Casebook of Midwifery and Obstetrical Nursing

(For BSc Nursing Students)

Casebook of Midwifery and Obstetrical Nursing

(For BSc Nursing Students)

Yasmin Mansoori
MSc Nursing (Obs & Gyn)
HOD
Obstetrics and Gynaecology Nursing
Mittal College of Nursing, Ajmer
Rajasthan, India

JAYPEE

JAYPEE BROTHERS MEDICAL PUBLISHERS
The Health Sciences Publisher
New Delhi | London

Jaypee Brothers Medical Publishers (P) Ltd

Headquarters
EMCA House
23/23-B, Ansari Road, Daryaganj
New Delhi 110 002, India
Landline: +91-11-23272143, +91-11-23272703
+91-11-23282021, +91-11-23245672
E-mail: jaypee@jaypeebrothers.comm

Corporate Office
4838/24, Ansari Road, Daryaganj
New Delhi 110 002, India
Phone: +91-11-43574357
Fax: +91-11-43574314
E-mail: jaypee@jaypeebrothers.com

Overseas Office
J.P. Medical Ltd.
83, Victoria Street, London
SW1H 0HW (UK)
Phone: +44-20 3170 8910
E-mail: info@jpmedpub.com

EU GPSR Authorised Representative
Logos Europe, 9 rue Nicolas Poussin
17000, La Rochelle, France
Phone: +33 (0) 6 67 93 73 78
E-mail: contact@logoseurope.eu

Website: www.jaypeebrothers.com
Website: www.jaypeedigital.com

Casebook of Midwifery and Obstetrical Nursing

First Edition: 2016

Reprint: **2026**

ISBN: 978-93-5152-993-4

Printed at: Samrat Offset Pvt. Ltd.

Dedicated to

My Family Members,
Teachers and Students

Preface

It gives me immense pleasure to present this 'Casebook of Midwifery and Obstetrical Nursing' for BSc Nursing Students.

This casebook is prepared as per Indian Nursing Council Syllabus, but it was most important opportunity as well as a challenge for me to provide all such content to undergraduate students in a simple manner, so that students could grasp the maximum information in a short time and correlate their theoretical knowledge into practical documentation to enhance their midwifery skill. I hope that the book will appeal to all nursing midwifery students as it fulfils their syllabus requirements.

It is indeed gratifying that this casebook would be helpful for clinical instructor to promote nursing students in achieving their midwifery skill.

Yasmin Mansoori

Acknowledgements

First of all I would like to thank the supreme power, the Almighty God, who has always guided me to work on the right path of life and without His grace this book 'Casebook of Midwifery and Obstetrical Nursing' would not have become reality.

I would like to express my gratitude to Dr Usha Uande (Principal, Choithram College of Nursing) for being so generous as to provide me guidance to achieve correct direction and for finding time for me in her busy schedule. Madam, words can never be enough to thank your kindness.

I would like to express my gratitude to all my teachers who put their faith in me and urged me to do better.

I also place on record, my sense of gratitude to one and all who directly and indirectly have lent their helping hands to finish the task.

I would also like to thank my parents, sisters, husband, family and friends who always motivated me to do new and fresh with full of energy and ideas, supporting me in all aspects.

The main motivating factor in writing this book was our students of midwifery who needed a practical knowledge in recording form.

I convey my sincere thanks to Jaypee Brothers Medical Publishers for their efforts and suggestions, especially Mr Jitendar P Vij (Group Chairman), Ms Chetna Vohra (Associate Director), and Ms Payal Bharti (Project Manager) for helping me through my idea. I also thank Mr Subrata Adhikary, Mr Aditya Singh, who persuaded me to take up the task of writing a book on midwifery casebook.

Student Record

Name of Student ....

....

Roll Number ....

Batch ....

Institution Name ....

....

Signature of Student *Signature of Class Coordinator* *Signature of Principal*

Essential Requirements

S.NO.	TITLE OF REQUIREMENTS	RECOMMENDED	COMPLETED
1.	Antenatal Examination	30	
2.	Intranatal Examination	20	
3.	Postnatal Examination	20	
4.	Vaginal Examination	05	
5.	Episiotomy and Suture	01	
6.	Neonatal Resuscitation	05	
7.	Assist with Caesarean Section	02	
8.	Witness/Assist Abnormal Deliveries	01	
9.	Insertion of IUD	05	

....

Signature of Internal Examiner *Signature of External Examiner*

....

Signature of Student *Signature of Class Coordinator* *Signature of Principal*

Contents

ANTENATAL EXAMINATION PERFORMED

S. No.	Date	Reg. No.	Name of the Patient	G, P, L, A	LMP	EDD	Wks of Gestation	Presentation/ Position	Baby Sex/Wt.	Supervised by
1.										
2.										
3.										
4.										
5.										
6.										
7.										
8.										
9.										
10.										
11.										
12.										
13.										
14.										
15.										
16.										
17.										
18.										
19.										
20.										
21.										
22.										
23.										
24.										
25.										
26.										
27.										
28.										
29.										
30.										

NORMAL DELIVERIES CONDUCTED

S. No.	Date	Reg. No.	Name of the Patient	G, P, L, A	LMP	EDD	Wks of Gestation	Presentation/ Position	Baby Sex/Wt.	Supervised by
1.										
2.										
3.										
4.										
5.										
6.										
7.										
8.										
9.										
10.										
11.										
12.										
13.										
14.										
15.										
16.										
17.										
18.										
19.										
20.										

POSTNATAL CARE PROVIDED

S.No	Date	Reg. No.	Name of the Patient	G, P, L, A	LMP	EDD	Wks of Gestation	Presentation/ Position	Baby Sex/ Wt.	Supervised by
1.										
2.										
3.										
4.										
5.										
6.										
7.										
8.										
9.										
10.										
11.										
12.										
13.										
14.										
15.										
16.										
17.										
18.										
19.										
20.										

VAGINAL EXAMINATION

S. No	Date	Reg. No.	Name of the Patient	G, P, L, A	LMP	EDD	Cervical Taken UP/ Dilatation	Membrane	Presentation/ Position	Indication
1.										
2.										
3.										
4.										
5.										

EPISIOTOMIES

S.No.	Date	Reg. No.	Name of the Patient	Gravida	Para	Indication	Type of Episiotomy	Remarks	Supervisor Signature
1.									
2.									
3.									
4.									
5.									

NEONATAL RESUSCITATION

S. No.	Date of Birth	Reg. No.	Name of the Pt./Baby	Time of Birth	Birth Weight	Mode of Delivery	Type of Labour	Apgar Score	Drug Given	Remark
1.										
2.										
3.										
4.										
5.										

ASSIST WITH CAESAREAN SECTION

S.No	Date	Reg. No.	Name of the Patient	G, P, L, A	LMP	EDD	Wks of Gestation	Presentation/ Position	Baby Sex/Wt.	Supervised by
1.										
2.										

WITNESS/ASSIST ABNORMAL DELIVERIES

S. No.	Date	Reg. No.	Name of the Patient	G, P, L, A	LMP	EDD	Wks of Gestation	Presentation/ Position	Baby Sex/Wt.	Supervised by
1.										
2.										
3.										
4.										
5.										

INSERTION OF IUD

S. No	Date	Reg. No.	Name of the Patient	G, P, L, A	Contraceptive used before	Last Menstrual Date	Choice of IUCD	Any Medical Problem	Remarks	Supervised by
1.										
2.										
3.										
4.										
5.										

ANTENATAL EXAMINATION

Name:________________ Age: ________ G, P, L, A ________________
Name of the Hospital:________________ Hospital Number: ________________
Date of Admission:________________ Weeks of Gestation:________________
Date of Registration:________ LMP: ________ EDD: ________________
High-risk Pregnancy Group: Yes/No

MEDICAL HISTORY

Chronic Illness:________________
Surgery:________________
Allergy:________________
Communicable Disease: ________________

FAMILY HISTORY

Type of Family:
Nuclear:________________ Number of persons:________________
Joint:________________ Number of persons: ________________

HISTORY OF MULTIPLE BIRTHS

Number of Children:________ Girl Child:________ Boy Child:________

SOCIOECONOMIC BACKGROUND

Religion:________________ Family Income:________________
Education: Husband: ________________ Wife: ________________
Occupation: Husband: ________________ Wife: ________________

MENSTRUAL HISTORY

Menarchy:________ Duration:________ Interval:________ Flow:________

MARITAL HISTORY

Age of Marriage:________________
Consanguineous: Yes/No

DIETARY PATTERN

Vegetarian:________________ Nonvegetarian: ________________
Likes:________________ Dislikes: ________________
Habits: Smoking/Drinking Alchohol/Chewing pan/Tobacco

HISTORY OF PREVIOUS PREGNANCIES

S. No.	Year	Full Term	Premature	Abortion	Mode of Delivery	Puerpe-rium	CHILD				
							Alive	Stillborn	Sex	Wt. at Birth	Growth and Develop

Diet Ordered: __________

Medications Ordered: __________

Treatment: __________

Remarks: __________

Nursing Intervention and Health Education:

PRENATAL VISITS

Date	Height	Weight	Urine	BP	FHR	Ht. of Fundus	Abd. Girth	Presenta-tion	Position	Treatment Remarks

GENERAL EXAMINATION

Date of Admission:__________ Diagnosis:__________

General condition: Good/Fair/Satisfactory/Poor

Heart: __________ Lungs:__________ Abdomen:__________

Breast:__________ Nipples:__________

Edema Ankles:__________ Hands:__________

TPR: __________ BP __________

Digestion: __________ Micturation: __________

Vaginal Discharge:__________

INVESTIGATION

Blood Group:__________ Rh Factor:__________ Hb:__________ VDRL:__________ HIV:__________

Others: __________

Ultrasonography: __________

REMARKS

Diet Ordered: __________

____

__________ Medication: __________

____

Nursing Interventions:__________

____

Health Education:__________

____

____

____

Sign of Supervisor **Sign of Student**

ANTENATAL EXAMINATION

Name:__________ Age: __________ G, P, L, A __________
Name of the Hospital:__________ Hospital Number: __________
Date of Admission:__________ Weeks of Gestation:__________
Date of Registration:__________ LMP: __________ EDD: __________
High-risk Pregnancy Group: Yes/No

MEDICAL HISTORY

Chronic Illness:__________
Surgery:__________
Allergy:__________
Communicable Disease: __________

FAMILY HISTORY

Type of Family:
Nuclear:__________ Number of persons:__________
Joint:__________ Number of persons: __________

HISTORY OF MULTIPLE BIRTHS

Number of Children:__________ Girl Child:__________ Boy Child:__________

SOCIOECONOMIC BACKGROUND

Religion:__________ Family Income:__________
Education: Husband: __________ Wife: __________
Occupation: Husband: __________ Wife: __________

MENSTRUAL HISTORY

Menarchy:__________ Duration:__________ Interval:__________ Flow:__________

MARITAL HISTORY

Age of Marriage:__________
Consanguineous: Yes/No

DIETARY PATTERN

Vegetarian:__________ Nonvegetarian: __________
Likes:__________ Dislikes: __________
Habits: Smoking/Drinking Alchohol/Chewing pan/Tobacco

HISTORY OF PREVIOUS PREGNANCIES

S. No.	Year	Full Term	Pre-mature	Abortion	Mode of Delivery	puerpe-rium	CHILD				
							Alive	Stillborn	Sex	Wt. at Birth	Growth and Develop

Diet Ordered:__________

Medications Ordered: __________

Treatment: __________

Remarks:__________

Nursing Intervention and Health Education:

PRENATAL VISITS

Date	Height	Weight	Urine	BP	FHR	Ht. of Fundus	Abd. Girth	Presenta-tion	Position	Treatment Remarks

GENERAL EXAMINATION

Date of Admission:__________ Diagnosis:__________

General condition: Good/Fair/Satisfactory/Poor

Heart: __________ Lungs:__________ Abdomen:__________

Breast:__________ Nipples:__________

Edema Ankles:__________ Hands:__________

TPR: __________ BP __________

Digestion: __________ Micturation: __________

Vaginal Discharge:__________

INVESTIGATION

Blood Group:__________ Rh Factor:__________ Hb:__________ VDRL:__________ HIV:__________

Others: __________

Ultrasonography: __________

REMARKS

Diet Ordered: __________

__________ Medication: __________

Nursing Interventions:__________

Health Education:__________

Sign of Supervisor **Sign of Student**

ANTENATAL EXAMINATION

Name:________________ Age: ________ G, P, L, A ________________
Name of the Hospital:________________ Hospital Number: ________________
Date of Admission:________________ Weeks of Gestation:________________
Date of Registration:__________ LMP: __________ EDD: ________________
High-risk Pregnancy Group: Yes/No

MEDICAL HISTORY

Chronic Illness:________________
Surgery:________________
Allergy:________________
Communicable Disease: ________________

FAMILY HISTORY

Type of Family:
Nuclear:________________ Number of persons:________________
Joint:________________ Number of persons: ________________

HISTORY OF MULTIPLE BIRTHS

Number of Children:__________ Girl Child:__________ Boy Child:__________

SOCIOECONOMIC BACKGROUND

Religion:________________ Family Income:________________
Education: Husband: ________________ Wife: ________________
Occupation: Husband: ________________ Wife: ________________

MENSTRUAL HISTORY

Menarchy:__________ Duration:__________ Interval:__________ Flow:__________

MARITAL HISTORY

Age of Marriage:________________
Consanguineous: Yes/No

DIETARY PATTERN

Vegetarian:________________ Nonvegetarian: ________________
Likes:________________ Dislikes: ________________
Habits: Smoking/Drinking Alchohol/Chewing pan/Tobacco

HISTORY OF PREVIOUS PREGNANCIES

S. No.	Year	Full Term	Pre-mature	Abortion	Mode of Delivery	puerpe-rium	CHILD				
							Alive	Stillborn	Sex	Wt. at Birth	Growth and Develop

Diet Ordered:____________________

Medications Ordered: ____________________

Treatment: ____________________

Remarks:____________________

Nursing Intervention and Health Education:

PRENATAL VISITS

Date	Height	Weight	Urine	BP	FHR	Ht. of Fundus	Abd. Girth	Presenta-tion	Position	Treatment Remarks

GENERAL EXAMINATION

Date of Admission:________________ Diagnosis:________________
General condition: Good/Fair/Satisfactory/Poor
Heart:__________ Lungs:__________ Abdomen:__________
Breast:__________ Nipples:__________
Edema Ankles:__________ Hands:__________
TPR:__________ BP__________
Digestion:__________ Micturation:__________
Vaginal Discharge:________________

INVESTIGATION

Blood Group:________ Rh Factor:________ Hb:________ VDRL:________ HIV:________
Others: ________________
Ultrasonography: ________________

REMARKS

Diet Ordered: ________________
____
________________ Medication: ________________
____

Nursing Interventions:________________
____

Health Education:________________
____
____
____

Sign of Supervisor **Sign of Student**

ANTENATAL EXAMINATION

Name:__________ Age: __________ G, P, L, A __________
Name of the Hospital:__________ Hospital Number: __________
Date of Admission:__________ Weeks of Gestation:__________
Date of Registration:__________ LMP: __________ EDD: __________
High-risk Pregnancy Group: Yes/No

MEDICAL HISTORY

Chronic Illness:__________
Surgery:__________
Allergy:__________
Communicable Disease: __________

FAMILY HISTORY

Type of Family:
Nuclear:__________ Number of persons:__________
Joint:__________ Number of persons: __________

HISTORY OF MULTIPLE BIRTHS

Number of Children:__________ Girl Child:__________ Boy Child:__________

SOCIOECONOMIC BACKGROUND

Religion:__________ Family Income:__________
Education: Husband: __________ Wife: __________
Occupation: Husband: __________ Wife: __________

MENSTRUAL HISTORY

Menarchy:__________ Duration:__________ Interval:__________ Flow:__________

MARITAL HISTORY

Age of Marriage:__________
Consanguineous: Yes/No

DIETARY PATTERN

Vegetarian:__________ Nonvegetarian: __________
Likes:__________ Dislikes: __________
Habits: Smoking/Drinking Alchohol/Chewing pan/Tobacco

HISTORY OF PREVIOUS PREGNANCIES

S. No.	Year	Full Term	Pre-mature	Abortion	Mode of Delivery	puerpe-rium	CHILD				
							Alive	Stillborn	Sex	Wt. at Birth	Growth and Develop

Diet Ordered:________________________________

Medications Ordered: ________________________________

Treatment: ________________________________

Remarks:________________________________

Nursing Intervention and Health Education:

PRENATAL VISITS

Date	Height	Weight	Urine	BP	FHR	Ht. of Fundus	Abd. Girth	Presenta-tion	Position	Treatment Remarks

GENERAL EXAMINATION

Date of Admission:________________ Diagnosis:________________

General condition: Good/Fair/Satisfactory/Poor

Heart: ________ Lungs:________ Abdomen:________

Breast:________Nipples:________

Edema Ankles:________Hands:________

TPR: ________ BP ________

Digestion: ________ Micturation: ________

Vaginal Discharge:________________

INVESTIGATION

Blood Group:________ Rh Factor:________ Hb:________ VDRL:________ HIV:________

Others: ________________

Ultrasonography: ________________

REMARKS

Diet Ordered: ________________

____

________________ Medication: ________________

____

Nursing Interventions:________________

____

Health Education:________________

____

____

____

Sign of Supervisor **Sign of Student**

ANTENATAL EXAMINATION

Name:_______________ Age: _______ G, P, L, A _______________
Name of the Hospital:_______________ Hospital Number: _______________
Date of Admission:_______________ Weeks of Gestation:_______________
Date of Registration:_________ LMP: _________ EDD: _______________
High-risk Pregnancy Group: Yes/No

MEDICAL HISTORY

Chronic Illness:_______________
Surgery:_______________
Allergy:_______________
Communicable Disease: _______________

FAMILY HISTORY

Type of Family:
Nuclear:_______________ Number of persons:_______________
Joint:_______________ Number of persons: _______________

HISTORY OF MULTIPLE BIRTHS

Number of Children:_________ Girl Child:_________ Boy Child:_________

SOCIOECONOMIC BACKGROUND

Religion:_______________ Family Income:_______________
Education: Husband: _______________ Wife: _______________
Occupation: Husband: _______________ Wife: _______________

MENSTRUAL HISTORY

Menarchy:_________ Duration:_________ Interval:_________ Flow:_________

MARITAL HISTORY

Age of Marriage:_______________
Consanguineous: Yes/No

DIETARY PATTERN

Vegetarian:_______________ Nonvegetarian: _______________
Likes:_______________ Dislikes: _______________
Habits: Smoking/Drinking Alchohol/Chewing pan/Tobacco

HISTORY OF PREVIOUS PREGNANCIES

S. No.	Year	Full Term	Pre-mature	Abortion	Mode of Delivery	puerpe-rium	CHILD				
							Alive	Stillborn	Sex	Wt. at Birth	Growth and Develop

Diet Ordered:____________________

Medications Ordered: ____________________

Treatment: ____________________

Remarks:____________________

Nursing Intervention and Health Education:

PRENATAL VISITS

Date	Height	Weight	Urine	BP	FHR	Ht. of Fundus	Abd. Girth	Presenta-tion	Position	Treatment Remarks

GENERAL EXAMINATION

Date of Admission:________________ Diagnosis:________________
General condition: Good/Fair/Satisfactory/Poor
Heart: ________ Lungs:________ Abdomen:________
Breast:________Nipples:________
Edema Ankles:________Hands:________
TPR: ________ BP ________
Digestion: ________ Micturation: ________
Vaginal Discharge:________

INVESTIGATION

Blood Group:________ Rh Factor:________ Hb:________ VDRL:________ HIV:________
Others: ________
Ultrasonography: ________

REMARKS

Diet Ordered: ________
____
________ Medication: ________
____

Nursing Interventions:________
____

Health Education:________
____
____
____

Sign of Supervisor **Sign of Student**

ANTENATAL EXAMINATION

Name:__________ Age: __________ G, P, L, A __________
Name of the Hospital:__________ Hospital Number: __________
Date of Admission:__________ Weeks of Gestation:__________
Date of Registration:__________ LMP: __________ EDD: __________
High-risk Pregnancy Group: Yes/No

MEDICAL HISTORY

Chronic Illness:__________
Surgery:__________
Allergy:__________
Communicable Disease: __________

FAMILY HISTORY

Type of Family:
Nuclear:__________ Number of persons:__________
Joint:__________ Number of persons: __________

HISTORY OF MULTIPLE BIRTHS

Number of Children:__________ Girl Child:__________ Boy Child:__________

SOCIOECONOMIC BACKGROUND

Religion:__________ Family Income:__________
Education: Husband: __________ Wife: __________
Occupation: Husband: __________ Wife: __________

MENSTRUAL HISTORY

Menarchy:__________ Duration:__________ Interval:__________ Flow:__________

MARITAL HISTORY

Age of Marriage:__________
Consanguineous: Yes/No

DIETARY PATTERN

Vegetarian:__________ Nonvegetarian: __________
Likes:__________ Dislikes: __________
Habits: Smoking/Drinking Alchohol/Chewing pan/Tobacco

HISTORY OF PREVIOUS PREGNANCIES

S. No.	Year	Full Term	Pre-mature	Abortion	Mode of Delivery	puerpe-rium	CHILD				
							Alive	Stillborn	Sex	Wt. at Birth	Growth and Develop

Diet Ordered:____________________

Medications Ordered: ____________________

Treatment: ____________________

Remarks:____________________

Nursing Intervention and Health Education:

PRENATAL VISITS

Date	Height	Weight	Urine	BP	FHR	Ht. of Fundus	Abd. Girth	Presenta-tion	Position	Treatment Remarks

GENERAL EXAMINATION

Date of Admission:________________ Diagnosis:________________

General condition: Good/Fair/Satisfactory/Poor

Heart: ____________ Lungs:____________ Abdomen:____________

Breast:________________Nipples:________________

Edema Ankles:________________Hands:________________

TPR: ________________ BP ________________

Digestion: ________________ Micturation: ________________

Vaginal Discharge:________________

INVESTIGATION

Blood Group:__________ Rh Factor:__________ Hb:__________ VDRL:__________ HIV:__________

Others: ________________

Ultrasonography: ________________

REMARKS

Diet Ordered: ________________

____

________________ Medication: ________________

____

Nursing Interventions:________________

____

Health Education:________________

____

____

____

Sign of Supervisor **Sign of Student**

ANTENATAL EXAMINATION

Name:__________ Age: __________ G, P, L, A __________
Name of the Hospital:__________ Hospital Number: __________
Date of Admission:__________ Weeks of Gestation:__________
Date of Registration:__________ LMP: __________ EDD: __________
High-risk Pregnancy Group: Yes/No

MEDICAL HISTORY

Chronic Illness:__________
Surgery:__________
Allergy:__________
Communicable Disease: __________

FAMILY HISTORY

Type of Family:
Nuclear:__________ Number of persons:__________
Joint:__________ Number of persons: __________

HISTORY OF MULTIPLE BIRTHS

Number of Children:__________ Girl Child:__________ Boy Child:__________

SOCIOECONOMIC BACKGROUND

Religion:__________ Family Income:__________
Education: Husband: __________ Wife: __________
Occupation: Husband: __________ Wife: __________

MENSTRUAL HISTORY

Menarchy:__________ Duration:__________ Interval:__________ Flow:__________

MARITAL HISTORY

Age of Marriage:__________
Consanguineous: Yes/No

DIETARY PATTERN

Vegetarian:__________ Nonvegetarian: __________
Likes:__________ Dislikes: __________
Habits: Smoking/Drinking Alchohol/Chewing pan/Tobacco

HISTORY OF PREVIOUS PREGNANCIES

S. No.	Year	Full Term	Pre-mature	Abortion	Mode of Delivery	puerpe-rium	CHILD				
							Alive	Stillborn	Sex	Wt. at Birth	Growth and Develop

Diet Ordered:____________________

Medications Ordered: ____________________

Treatment: ____________________

Remarks:____________________

Nursing Intervention and Health Education:

PRENATAL VISITS

Date	Height	Weight	Urine	BP	FHR	Ht. of Fundus	Abd. Girth	Presenta-tion	Position	Treatment Remarks

GENERAL EXAMINATION

Date of Admission:________________________ Diagnosis:________________________

General condition: Good/Fair/Satisfactory/Poor

Heart: ____________ Lungs:________________ Abdomen:________________

Breast:________________Nipples:________________________

Edema Ankles:____________________Hands:____________________

TPR: ________________________ BP ____________________

Digestion: ____________________ Micturation: ____________________

Vaginal Discharge:____

INVESTIGATION

Blood Group:__________ Rh Factor:________ Hb:________ VDRL:________ HIV:________

Others: ____

Ultrasonography: ____

REMARKS

Diet Ordered: ____

____

____________________ Medication: ____________________

____

Nursing Interventions:____

____

Health Education:____

____

____

____

Sign of Supervisor **Sign of Student**

ANTENATAL EXAMINATION

Name:________________________ Age: ______________ G, P, L, A ______________________
Name of the Hospital:_____________________ Hospital Number: ____________________
Date of Admission:_______________________ Weeks of Gestation:___________________
Date of Registration:______________ LMP: ______________ EDD: ____________________
High-risk Pregnancy Group: Yes/No

MEDICAL HISTORY

Chronic Illness:____
Surgery:____
Allergy:____
Communicable Disease: ____

–

FAMILY HISTORY

Type of Family:
Nuclear:_______________________________ Number of persons:____________________
Joint:_______________________________ Number of persons: _____________________

–

HISTORY OF MULTIPLE BIRTHS

Number of Children:___________________ Girl Child:_______________ Boy Child:_______________

SOCIOECONOMIC BACKGROUND

Religion:____________________________________ Family Income:_____________________
Education: Husband: _____________________________ Wife: ___________________________
Occupation: Husband: ___________________________ Wife: ____________________________

MENSTRUAL HISTORY

Menarchy:________________ Duration:______________ Interval:______________ Flow:__________

MARITAL HISTORY

Age of Marriage:______________________________
Consanguineous: Yes/No

DIETARY PATTERN

Vegetarian:_______________________________ Nonvegetarian: ________________________
Likes:___________________________________ Dislikes: ____________________________
Habits: Smoking/Drinking Alchohol/Chewing pan/Tobacco

HISTORY OF PREVIOUS PREGNANCIES

S. No.	Year	Full Term	Pre-mature	Abortion	Mode of Delivery	puerpe-rium	CHILD				
							Alive	Stillborn	Sex	Wt. at Birth	Growth and Develop

Diet Ordered:__________

Medications Ordered: __________

Treatment: __________

Remarks:__________

Nursing Intervention and Health Education:

PRENATAL VISITS

Date	Height	Weight	Urine	BP	FHR	Ht. of Fundus	Abd. Girth	Presenta-tion	Position	Treatment Remarks

GENERAL EXAMINATION

Date of Admission:______________________ Diagnosis:______________________
General condition: Good/Fair/Satisfactory/Poor
Heart:__________ Lungs:______________ Abdomen:______________
Breast:______________ Nipples:______________________
Edema Ankles:______________________ Hands:______________
TPR:______________________ BP______________
Digestion:______________________ Micturation:______________
Vaginal Discharge:______________________________________

INVESTIGATION

Blood Group:__________ Rh Factor:__________ Hb:__________ VDRL:__________ HIV:__________
Others: ______________________________________
Ultrasonography: ______________________________________

REMARKS

Diet Ordered: ______________________________________

______________________ Medication: ______________________

Nursing Interventions:______________________________________

Health Education:______________________________________

Sign of Supervisor **Sign of Student**

ANTENATAL EXAMINATION

Name:________________ Age: ________ G, P, L, A ________________
Name of the Hospital:________________ Hospital Number: ________________
Date of Admission:________________ Weeks of Gestation:________________
Date of Registration:__________ LMP: __________ EDD: ________________
High-risk Pregnancy Group: Yes/No

MEDICAL HISTORY

Chronic Illness:________________________________
Surgery:________________________________
Allergy:________________________________
Communicable Disease: ________________________________

FAMILY HISTORY

Type of Family:
Nuclear:________________ Number of persons:________________
Joint:________________ Number of persons: ________________

HISTORY OF MULTIPLE BIRTHS

Number of Children:__________ Girl Child:__________ Boy Child:__________

SOCIOECONOMIC BACKGROUND

Religion:________________ Family Income:________________
Education: Husband: ________________ Wife: ________________
Occupation: Husband: ________________ Wife: ________________

MENSTRUAL HISTORY

Menarchy:__________ Duration:__________ Interval:__________ Flow:__________

MARITAL HISTORY

Age of Marriage:________________
Consanguineous: Yes/No

DIETARY PATTERN

Vegetarian:________________ Nonvegetarian: ________________
Likes:________________ Dislikes: ________________
Habits: Smoking/Drinking Alchohol/Chewing pan/Tobacco

HISTORY OF PREVIOUS PREGNANCIES

S. No.	Year	Full Term	Pre-mature	Abortion	Mode of Delivery	puerpe-rium	CHILD				
							Alive	Stillborn	Sex	Wt. at Birth	Growth and Develop

Diet Ordered: ____________________

Medications Ordered: ____________________

____

Treatment: ____________________

____

Remarks: ____________________

Nursing Intervention and Health Education:

____

____

____

____

____

____

____

____

____

____

____

PRENATAL VISITS

Date	Height	Weight	Urine	BP	FHR	Ht. of Fundus	Abd. Girth	Presenta-tion	Position	Treatment Remarks

GENERAL EXAMINATION

Date of Admission:____________________ Diagnosis:____________________
General condition: Good/Fair/Satisfactory/Poor
Heart: __________ Lungs:__________ Abdomen:__________
Breast:__________Nipples:__________
Edema Ankles:__________Hands:__________
TPR: __________ BP __________
Digestion: __________ Micturation: __________
Vaginal Discharge:__________

INVESTIGATION

Blood Group:__________ Rh Factor:__________ Hb:__________ VDRL:__________ HIV:__________
Others: __________
Ultrasonography: __________

REMARKS

Diet Ordered: __________
____
__________ Medication: __________
____

Nursing Interventions:__________
____

Health Education:__________
____
____
____

Sign of Supervisor **Sign of Student**

ANTENATAL EXAMINATION

Name:__________ Age: __________ G, P, L, A __________
Name of the Hospital:__________ Hospital Number: __________
Date of Admission:__________ Weeks of Gestation:__________
Date of Registration:__________ LMP: __________ EDD: __________
High-risk Pregnancy Group: Yes/No

MEDICAL HISTORY

Chronic Illness:__________
Surgery:__________
Allergy:__________
Communicable Disease: __________

FAMILY HISTORY

Type of Family:
Nuclear:__________ Number of persons:__________
Joint:__________ Number of persons: __________

HISTORY OF MULTIPLE BIRTHS

Number of Children:__________ Girl Child:__________ Boy Child:__________

SOCIOECONOMIC BACKGROUND

Religion:__________ Family Income:__________
Education: Husband: __________ Wife: __________
Occupation: Husband: __________ Wife: __________

MENSTRUAL HISTORY

Menarchy:__________ Duration:__________ Interval:__________ Flow:__________

MARITAL HISTORY

Age of Marriage:__________
Consanguineous: Yes/No

DIETARY PATTERN

Vegetarian:__________ Nonvegetarian: __________
Likes:__________ Dislikes: __________
Habits: Smoking/Drinking Alchohol/Chewing pan/Tobacco

HISTORY OF PREVIOUS PREGNANCIES

S. No.	Year	Full Term	Pre-mature	Abortion	Mode of Delivery	puerpe-rium	CHILD				
							Alive	Stillborn	Sex	Wt. at Birth	Growth and Develop

Diet Ordered: __________

Medications Ordered: __________

Treatment: __________

Remarks: __________

Nursing Intervention and Health Education:

PRENATAL VISITS

Date	Height	Weight	Urine	BP	FHR	Ht. of Fundus	Abd. Girth	Presenta-tion	Position	Treatment Remarks

GENERAL EXAMINATION

Date of Admission:________________________ Diagnosis:________________________

General condition: Good/Fair/Satisfactory/Poor

Heart: ____________ Lungs:________________ Abdomen:________________

Breast:________________ Nipples:________________________

Edema Ankles:________________________ Hands:________________

TPR: ________________________ BP ________________

Digestion: ________________ Micturation: ________________

Vaginal Discharge:____

INVESTIGATION

Blood Group:__________ Rh Factor:________ Hb:________ VDRL:________ HIV:________

Others: ____

Ultrasonography: ____

REMARKS

Diet Ordered: ____

____

________________ Medication: ________________________

____

Nursing Interventions:____

____

Health Education:____

____

____

____

Sign of Supervisor **Sign of Student**

ANTENATAL EXAMINATION

Name:__________ Age: __________ G, P, L, A __________
Name of the Hospital:__________ Hospital Number: __________
Date of Admission:__________ Weeks of Gestation:__________
Date of Registration:__________ LMP: __________ EDD: __________
High-risk Pregnancy Group: Yes/No

MEDICAL HISTORY

Chronic Illness:__________
Surgery:__________
Allergy:__________
Communicable Disease: __________

FAMILY HISTORY

Type of Family:
Nuclear:__________ Number of persons:__________
Joint:__________ Number of persons: __________

HISTORY OF MULTIPLE BIRTHS

Number of Children:__________ Girl Child:__________ Boy Child:__________

SOCIOECONOMIC BACKGROUND

Religion:__________ Family Income:__________
Education: Husband: __________ Wife: __________
Occupation: Husband: __________ Wife: __________

MENSTRUAL HISTORY

Menarchy:__________ Duration:__________ Interval:__________ Flow:__________

MARITAL HISTORY

Age of Marriage:__________
Consanguineous: Yes/No

DIETARY PATTERN

Vegetarian:__________ Nonvegetarian: __________
Likes:__________ Dislikes: __________
Habits: Smoking/Drinking Alchohol/Chewing pan/Tobacco

HISTORY OF PREVIOUS PREGNANCIES

S. No.	Year	Full Term	Pre-mature	Abortion	Mode of Delivery	puerpe-rium	CHILD				
							Alive	Stillborn	Sex	Wt. at Birth	Growth and Develop

Diet Ordered: ____________________

Medications Ordered: ____________________

Treatment: ____________________

Remarks: ____________________

Nursing Intervention and Health Education:

PRENATAL VISITS

Date	Height	Weight	Urine	BP	FHR	Ht. of Fundus	Abd. Girth	Presenta-tion	Position	Treatment Remarks

GENERAL EXAMINATION

Date of Admission:__________ Diagnosis:__________

General condition: Good/Fair/Satisfactory/Poor

Heart: __________ Lungs:__________ Abdomen:__________

Breast:__________ Nipples:__________

Edema Ankles:__________ Hands:__________

TPR: __________ BP __________

Digestion: __________ Micturation: __________

Vaginal Discharge:__________

INVESTIGATION

Blood Group:__________ Rh Factor:__________ Hb:__________ VDRL:__________ HIV:__________

Others: __________

Ultrasonography: __________

REMARKS

Diet Ordered: __________

__________ Medication: __________

Nursing Interventions:__________

Health Education:__________

Sign of Supervisor **Sign of Student**

ANTENATAL EXAMINATION

Name:________________ Age: ________ G, P, L, A ________________
Name of the Hospital:________________ Hospital Number: ________________
Date of Admission:________________ Weeks of Gestation:________________
Date of Registration:__________ LMP: __________ EDD: ________________
High-risk Pregnancy Group: Yes/No

MEDICAL HISTORY

Chronic Illness:________________
Surgery:________________
Allergy:________________
Communicable Disease: ________________

FAMILY HISTORY

Type of Family:
Nuclear:________________ Number of persons:________________
Joint:________________ Number of persons: ________________

HISTORY OF MULTIPLE BIRTHS

Number of Children:__________ Girl Child:__________ Boy Child:__________

SOCIOECONOMIC BACKGROUND

Religion:________________ Family Income:________________
Education: Husband: ________________ Wife: ________________
Occupation: Husband: ________________ Wife: ________________

MENSTRUAL HISTORY

Menarchy:__________ Duration:__________ Interval:__________ Flow:__________

MARITAL HISTORY

Age of Marriage:________________
Consanguineous: Yes/No

DIETARY PATTERN

Vegetarian:________________ Nonvegetarian: ________________
Likes:________________ Dislikes: ________________
Habits: Smoking/Drinking Alchohol/Chewing pan/Tobacco

HISTORY OF PREVIOUS PREGNANCIES

S. No.	Year	Full Term	Pre-mature	Abortion	Mode of Delivery	puerpe-rium	CHILD				
							Alive	Stillborn	Sex	Wt. at Birth	Growth and Develop

Diet Ordered:

Medications Ordered:

Treatment:

Remarks:

Nursing Intervention and Health Education:

PRENATAL VISITS

Date	Height	Weight	Urine	BP	FHR	Ht. of Fundus	Abd. Girth	Presenta-tion	Position	Treatment Remarks

GENERAL EXAMINATION

Date of Admission:________________ Diagnosis:________________
General condition: Good/Fair/Satisfactory/Poor
Heart: ________ Lungs:________ Abdomen:________
Breast:________________Nipples:________________
Edema Ankles:________________Hands:________________
TPR: ________________ BP ________________
Digestion: ________________ Micturation: ________________
Vaginal Discharge:________________

INVESTIGATION

Blood Group:________ Rh Factor:________ Hb:________ VDRL:________ HIV:________
Others: ________________
Ultrasonography: ________________

REMARKS

Diet Ordered: ________________
____
________________ Medication: ________________
____

Nursing Interventions:________________
____

Health Education:________________
____
____
____

Sign of Supervisor **Sign of Student**

ANTENATAL EXAMINATION

Name:________________ Age: ________ G, P, L, A ________________
Name of the Hospital:________________ Hospital Number: ________________
Date of Admission:________________ Weeks of Gestation:________________
Date of Registration:__________ LMP: __________ EDD: ________________
High-risk Pregnancy Group: Yes/No

MEDICAL HISTORY

Chronic Illness:________________
Surgery:________________
Allergy:________________
Communicable Disease: ________________

FAMILY HISTORY

Type of Family:
Nuclear:________________ Number of persons:________________
Joint:________________ Number of persons: ________________

HISTORY OF MULTIPLE BIRTHS

Number of Children:__________ Girl Child:__________ Boy Child:__________

SOCIOECONOMIC BACKGROUND

Religion:________________ Family Income:________________
Education: Husband: ________________ Wife: ________________
Occupation: Husband: ________________ Wife: ________________

MENSTRUAL HISTORY

Menarchy:__________ Duration:__________ Interval:__________ Flow:__________

MARITAL HISTORY

Age of Marriage:________________
Consanguineous: Yes/No

DIETARY PATTERN

Vegetarian:________________ Nonvegetarian: ________________
Likes:________________ Dislikes: ________________
Habits: Smoking/Drinking Alchohol/Chewing pan/Tobacco

HISTORY OF PREVIOUS PREGNANCIES

S. No.	Year	Full Term	Pre-mature	Abortion	Mode of Delivery	puerpe-rium	CHILD				
							Alive	Stillborn	Sex	Wt. at Birth	Growth and Develop

Diet Ordered: __________

Medications Ordered: __________

Treatment: __________

Remarks: __________

Nursing Intervention and Health Education:

PRENATAL VISITS

Date	Height	Weight	Urine	BP	FHR	Ht. of Fundus	Abd. Girth	Presenta-tion	Position	Treatment Remarks

GENERAL EXAMINATION

Date of Admission:__________ Diagnosis:__________
General condition: Good/Fair/Satisfactory/Poor
Heart: __________ Lungs:__________ Abdomen:__________
Breast:__________Nipples:__________
Edema Ankles:__________Hands:__________
TPR: __________ BP __________
Digestion: __________ Micturation: __________
Vaginal Discharge:__________

INVESTIGATION

Blood Group:__________ Rh Factor:__________ Hb:__________ VDRL:__________ HIV:__________
Others: __________
Ultrasonography: __________

REMARKS

Diet Ordered: __________
____
__________ Medication: __________
____

Nursing Interventions:__________
____

Health Education:__________
____
____
____

Sign of Supervisor **Sign of Student**

ANTENATAL EXAMINATION

Name:________________ Age: ________ G, P, L, A ________________
Name of the Hospital:________________ Hospital Number: ________________
Date of Admission:________________ Weeks of Gestation:________________
Date of Registration:________ LMP: ________ EDD: ________________
High-risk Pregnancy Group: Yes/No

MEDICAL HISTORY

Chronic Illness:________________
Surgery:________________
Allergy:________________
Communicable Disease: ________________

FAMILY HISTORY

Type of Family:
Nuclear:________________ Number of persons:________________
Joint:________________ Number of persons: ________________

HISTORY OF MULTIPLE BIRTHS

Number of Children:________ Girl Child:________ Boy Child:________

SOCIOECONOMIC BACKGROUND

Religion:________________ Family Income:________________
Education: Husband: ________________ Wife: ________________
Occupation: Husband: ________________ Wife: ________________

MENSTRUAL HISTORY

Menarchy:________ Duration:________ Interval:________ Flow:________

MARITAL HISTORY

Age of Marriage:________________
Consanguineous: Yes/No

DIETARY PATTERN

Vegetarian:________________ Nonvegetarian: ________________
Likes:________________ Dislikes: ________________
Habits: Smoking/Drinking Alchohol/Chewing pan/Tobacco

HISTORY OF PREVIOUS PREGNANCIES

S. No.	Year	Full Term	Pre-mature	Abortion	Mode of Delivery	puerpe-rium	CHILD				
							Alive	Stillborn	Sex	Wt. at Birth	Growth and Develop

Diet Ordered:__________

Medications Ordered: __________

Treatment: __________

Remarks:__________

Nursing Intervention and Health Education:

PRENATAL VISITS

Date	Height	Weight	Urine	BP	FHR	Ht. of Fundus	Abd. Girth	Presenta-tion	Position	Treatment Remarks

GENERAL EXAMINATION

Date of Admission:____ Diagnosis:____
General condition: Good/Fair/Satisfactory/Poor
Heart: ____ Lungs:____ Abdomen:____
Breast:____ Nipples:____
Edema Ankles:____ Hands:____
TPR: ____ BP ____
Digestion: ____ Micturation: ____
Vaginal Discharge:____

INVESTIGATION

Blood Group:____ Rh Factor:____ Hb:____ VDRL:____ HIV:____
Others: ____
Ultrasonography: ____

REMARKS

Diet Ordered: ____

____ Medication: ____

Nursing Interventions:____

Health Education:____

Sign of Supervisor **Sign of Student**

ANTENATAL EXAMINATION

Name:________________ Age: ________ G, P, L, A ________________
Name of the Hospital:________________ Hospital Number: ________________
Date of Admission:________________ Weeks of Gestation:________________
Date of Registration:__________ LMP: __________ EDD: ________________
High-risk Pregnancy Group: Yes/No

MEDICAL HISTORY

Chronic Illness:________________
Surgery:________________
Allergy:________________
Communicable Disease: ________________

FAMILY HISTORY

Type of Family:
Nuclear:________________ Number of persons:________________
Joint:________________ Number of persons: ________________

HISTORY OF MULTIPLE BIRTHS

Number of Children:__________ Girl Child:__________ Boy Child:__________

SOCIOECONOMIC BACKGROUND

Religion:________________ Family Income:________________
Education: Husband: ________________ Wife: ________________
Occupation: Husband: ________________ Wife: ________________

MENSTRUAL HISTORY

Menarchy:__________ Duration:__________ Interval:__________ Flow:__________

MARITAL HISTORY

Age of Marriage:________________
Consanguineous: Yes/No

DIETARY PATTERN

Vegetarian:________________ Nonvegetarian: ________________
Likes:________________ Dislikes: ________________
Habits: Smoking/Drinking Alchohol/Chewing pan/Tobacco

HISTORY OF PREVIOUS PREGNANCIES

S. No.	Year	Full Term	Pre-mature	Abortion	Mode of Delivery	puerpe-rium	CHILD				
							Alive	Stillborn	Sex	Wt. at Birth	Growth and Develop

Diet Ordered:

Medications Ordered:

Treatment:

Remarks:

Nursing Intervention and Health Education:

PRENATAL VISITS

Date	Height	Weight	Urine	BP	FHR	Ht. of Fundus	Abd. Girth	Presenta-tion	Position	Treatment Remarks

GENERAL EXAMINATION

Date of Admission:__________ Diagnosis:__________

General condition: Good/Fair/Satisfactory/Poor

Heart: __________ Lungs:__________ Abdomen:__________

Breast:__________Nipples:__________

Edema Ankles:__________Hands:__________

TPR: __________ BP __________

Digestion: __________ Micturation: __________

Vaginal Discharge:__________

INVESTIGATION

Blood Group:__________ Rh Factor:__________ Hb:__________ VDRL:__________ HIV:__________

Others: __________

Ultrasonography: __________

REMARKS

Diet Ordered: __________

____

__________ Medication: __________

____

Nursing Interventions:__________

____

Health Education:__________

____

____

____

Sign of Supervisor **Sign of Student**

ANTENATAL EXAMINATION

Name:________________ Age: ________ G, P, L, A ________________
Name of the Hospital:________________ Hospital Number: ________________
Date of Admission:________________ Weeks of Gestation:________________
Date of Registration:__________ LMP: __________ EDD: ________________
High-risk Pregnancy Group: Yes/No

MEDICAL HISTORY

Chronic Illness:________________
Surgery:________________
Allergy:________________
Communicable Disease: ________________

FAMILY HISTORY

Type of Family:
Nuclear:________________ Number of persons:________________
Joint:________________ Number of persons: ________________

HISTORY OF MULTIPLE BIRTHS

Number of Children:__________ Girl Child:__________ Boy Child:__________

SOCIOECONOMIC BACKGROUND

Religion:________________ Family Income:________________
Education: Husband: ________________ Wife: ________________
Occupation: Husband: ________________ Wife: ________________

MENSTRUAL HISTORY

Menarchy:__________ Duration:__________ Interval:__________ Flow:__________

MARITAL HISTORY

Age of Marriage:________________
Consanguineous: Yes/No

DIETARY PATTERN

Vegetarian:________________ Nonvegetarian: ________________
Likes:________________ Dislikes: ________________
Habits: Smoking/Drinking Alchohol/Chewing pan/Tobacco

HISTORY OF PREVIOUS PREGNANCIES

S. No.	Year	Full Term	Pre-mature	Abortion	Mode of Delivery	puerpe-rium	CHILD				
							Alive	Stillborn	Sex	Wt. at Birth	Growth and Develop

Diet Ordered:__________

Medications Ordered: __________

Treatment: __________

Remarks:__________

Nursing Intervention and Health Education:

PRENATAL VISITS

Date	Height	Weight	Urine	BP	FHR	Ht. of Fundus	Abd. Girth	Presenta-tion	Position	Treatment Remarks

GENERAL EXAMINATION

Date of Admission:________________ Diagnosis:________________

General condition: Good/Fair/Satisfactory/Poor

Heart: ____________ Lungs:________________ Abdomen:________________

Breast:________________Nipples:________________

Edema Ankles:________________Hands:________________

TPR: ________________ BP ________________

Digestion: ________________ Micturation: ________________

Vaginal Discharge:________________

INVESTIGATION

Blood Group:__________ Rh Factor:________ Hb:________ VDRL:________ HIV:________

Others: ________________

Ultrasonography: ________________

REMARKS

Diet Ordered: ________________

____

________________ Medication: ________________

____

Nursing Interventions:________________

____

Health Education:________________

____

____

____

Sign of Supervisor **Sign of Student**

ANTENATAL EXAMINATION

Name:________________ Age: ________ G, P, L, A ________________
Name of the Hospital:________________ Hospital Number: ________________
Date of Admission:________________ Weeks of Gestation:________________
Date of Registration:__________ LMP: __________ EDD: ________________
High-risk Pregnancy Group: Yes/No

MEDICAL HISTORY

Chronic Illness:________________________________
Surgery:________________________________
Allergy:________________________________
Communicable Disease: ________________________________

FAMILY HISTORY

Type of Family:
Nuclear:________________ Number of persons:________________
Joint:________________ Number of persons: ________________

HISTORY OF MULTIPLE BIRTHS

Number of Children:__________ Girl Child:__________ Boy Child:__________

SOCIOECONOMIC BACKGROUND

Religion:________________ Family Income:________________
Education: Husband: ________________ Wife: ________________
Occupation: Husband: ________________ Wife: ________________

MENSTRUAL HISTORY

Menarchy:__________ Duration:__________ Interval:__________ Flow:__________

MARITAL HISTORY

Age of Marriage:________________
Consanguineous: Yes/No

DIETARY PATTERN

Vegetarian:________________ Nonvegetarian: ________________
Likes:________________ Dislikes: ________________
Habits: Smoking/Drinking Alchohol/Chewing pan/Tobacco

HISTORY OF PREVIOUS PREGNANCIES

S. No.	Year	Full Term	Pre-mature	Abortion	Mode of Delivery	puerpe-rium	CHILD				
							Alive	Stillborn	Sex	Wt. at Birth	Growth and Develop

Diet Ordered:____________________

Medications Ordered: ____________________

____

Treatment: ____________________

____

Remarks:____________________

Nursing Intervention and Health Education:

____

____

____

____

____

____

____

____

____

____

____

PRENATAL VISITS

Date	Height	Weight	Urine	BP	FHR	Ht. of Fundus	Abd. Girth	Presenta-tion	Position	Treatment Remarks

GENERAL EXAMINATION

Date of Admission:_______________ Diagnosis:_______________
General condition: Good/Fair/Satisfactory/Poor
Heart: _______________ Lungs:_______________ Abdomen:_______________
Breast:_______________ Nipples:_______________
Edema Ankles:_______________ Hands:_______________
TPR: _______________ BP _______________
Digestion: _______________ Micturation: _______________
Vaginal Discharge:_______________

INVESTIGATION

Blood Group:_______________ Rh Factor:_______________ Hb:_______________ VDRL:_______________ HIV:_______________
Others: _______________
Ultrasonography: _______________

REMARKS

Diet Ordered: _______________
____
_______________ Medication: _______________
____

Nursing Interventions:_______________
____

Health Education:_______________
____
____
____

Sign of Supervisor **Sign of Student**

ANTENATAL EXAMINATION

Name:__________ Age: __________ G, P, L, A __________
Name of the Hospital:__________ Hospital Number: __________
Date of Admission:__________ Weeks of Gestation:__________
Date of Registration:__________ LMP: __________ EDD: __________
High-risk Pregnancy Group: Yes/No

MEDICAL HISTORY

Chronic Illness:__________
Surgery:__________
Allergy:__________
Communicable Disease: __________

FAMILY HISTORY

Type of Family:
Nuclear:__________ Number of persons:__________
Joint:__________ Number of persons: __________

HISTORY OF MULTIPLE BIRTHS

Number of Children:__________ Girl Child:__________ Boy Child:__________

SOCIOECONOMIC BACKGROUND

Religion:__________ Family Income:__________
Education: Husband: __________ Wife: __________
Occupation: Husband: __________ Wife: __________

MENSTRUAL HISTORY

Menarchy:__________ Duration:__________ Interval:__________ Flow:__________

MARITAL HISTORY

Age of Marriage:__________
Consanguineous: Yes/No

DIETARY PATTERN

Vegetarian:__________ Nonvegetarian: __________
Likes:__________ Dislikes: __________
Habits: Smoking/Drinking Alchohol/Chewing pan/Tobacco

HISTORY OF PREVIOUS PREGNANCIES

S. No.	Year	Full Term	Pre-mature	Abortion	Mode of Delivery	puerpe-rium	CHILD				
							Alive	Stillborn	Sex	Wt. at Birth	Growth and Develop

Diet Ordered:____________________

Medications Ordered: ____________________

Treatment: ____________________

Remarks:____________________

Nursing Intervention and Health Education:

PRENATAL VISITS

Date	Height	Weight	Urine	BP	FHR	Ht. of Fundus	Abd. Girth	Presenta-tion	Position	Treatment Remarks

GENERAL EXAMINATION

Date of Admission:________________ Diagnosis:________________

General condition: Good/Fair/Satisfactory/Poor

Heart: __________ Lungs:__________ Abdomen:__________

Breast:________________Nipples:________________

Edema Ankles:________________Hands:________________

TPR: ________________ BP ________________

Digestion: ________________ Micturation: ________________

Vaginal Discharge:________________

INVESTIGATION

Blood Group:________ Rh Factor:________ Hb:________ VDRL:________ HIV:________

Others: ________________

Ultrasonography: ________________

REMARKS

Diet Ordered: ________________

____

________________ Medication: ________________

____

Nursing Interventions:________________

____

Health Education:________________

____

____

____

Sign of Supervisor **Sign of Student**

ANTENATAL EXAMINATION

Name:______ Age: ______ G, P, L, A ______
Name of the Hospital:______ Hospital Number: ______
Date of Admission:______ Weeks of Gestation:______
Date of Registration:______ LMP: ______ EDD: ______
High-risk Pregnancy Group: Yes/No

MEDICAL HISTORY

Chronic Illness:______
Surgery:______
Allergy:______
Communicable Disease: ______

FAMILY HISTORY

Type of Family:
Nuclear:______ Number of persons:______
Joint:______ Number of persons: ______

HISTORY OF MULTIPLE BIRTHS

Number of Children:______ Girl Child:______ Boy Child:______

SOCIOECONOMIC BACKGROUND

Religion:______ Family Income:______
Education: Husband: ______ Wife: ______
Occupation: Husband: ______ Wife: ______

MENSTRUAL HISTORY

Menarchy:______ Duration:______ Interval:______ Flow:______

MARITAL HISTORY

Age of Marriage:______
Consanguineous: Yes/No

DIETARY PATTERN

Vegetarian:______ Nonvegetarian: ______
Likes:______ Dislikes: ______
Habits: Smoking/Drinking Alchohol/Chewing pan/Tobacco

HISTORY OF PREVIOUS PREGNANCIES

S. No.	Year	Full Term	Pre-mature	Abortion	Mode of Delivery	puerpe-rium	CHILD				
							Alive	Stillborn	Sex	Wt. at Birth	Growth and Develop

Diet Ordered: ____________________

Medications Ordered: ____________________

____

Treatment: ____________________

____

Remarks: ____________________

Nursing Intervention and Health Education:

____

____

____

____

____

____

____

____

____

____

____

PRENATAL VISITS

Date	Height	Weight	Urine	BP	FHR	Ht. of Fundus	Abd. Girth	Presenta-tion	Position	Treatment Remarks

GENERAL EXAMINATION

Date of Admission:____________________ Diagnosis:____________________

General condition: Good/Fair/Satisfactory/Poor

Heart: __________ Lungs:__________ Abdomen:__________

Breast:__________Nipples:__________

Edema Ankles:__________Hands:__________

TPR: __________ BP __________

Digestion: __________ Micturation: __________

Vaginal Discharge:__________

INVESTIGATION

Blood Group:________ Rh Factor:________ Hb:________ VDRL:________ HIV:________

Others: __________

Ultrasonography: __________

REMARKS

Diet Ordered: __________

__________ Medication: __________

Nursing Interventions:__________

Health Education:__________

Sign of Supervisor **Sign of Student**

ANTENATAL EXAMINATION

Name:_____ Age: _____ G, P, L, A _____
Name of the Hospital:_____ Hospital Number: _____
Date of Admission:_____ Weeks of Gestation:_____
Date of Registration:_____ LMP: _____ EDD: _____
High-risk Pregnancy Group: Yes/No

MEDICAL HISTORY

Chronic Illness:_____
Surgery:_____
Allergy:_____
Communicable Disease: _____

FAMILY HISTORY

Type of Family:
Nuclear:_____ Number of persons:_____
Joint:_____ Number of persons: _____

HISTORY OF MULTIPLE BIRTHS

Number of Children:_____ Girl Child:_____ Boy Child:_____

SOCIOECONOMIC BACKGROUND

Religion:_____ Family Income:_____
Education: Husband: _____ Wife: _____
Occupation: Husband: _____ Wife: _____

MENSTRUAL HISTORY

Menarchy:_____ Duration:_____ Interval:_____ Flow:_____

MARITAL HISTORY

Age of Marriage:_____
Consanguineous: Yes/No

DIETARY PATTERN

Vegetarian:_____ Nonvegetarian: _____
Likes:_____ Dislikes: _____
Habits: Smoking/Drinking Alchohol/Chewing pan/Tobacco

HISTORY OF PREVIOUS PREGNANCIES

S. No.	Year	Full Term	Pre-mature	Abortion	Mode of Delivery	puerpe-rium	CHILD				
							Alive	Stillborn	Sex	Wt. at Birth	Growth and Develop

Diet Ordered: ___

Medications Ordered: ___

___

Treatment: ___

___

Remarks: ___

Nursing Intervention and Health Education:

___

___

___

___

___

___

___

___

___

___

___

PRENATAL VISITS

Date	Height	Weight	Urine	BP	FHR	Ht. of Fundus	Abd. Girth	Presenta-tion	Position	Treatment Remarks

GENERAL EXAMINATION

Date of Admission:______________________________ Diagnosis:______________________________

General condition: Good/Fair/Satisfactory/Poor

Heart: ______________ Lungs:______________________ Abdomen:______________________

Breast:______________________Nipples:______________________________________

Edema Ankles:______________________________Hands:______________________________

TPR: ______________________________________ BP ______________________________

Digestion: ______________________________ Micturation: ______________________________

Vaginal Discharge:____

INVESTIGATION

Blood Group:______________ Rh Factor:__________ Hb:__________ VDRL:__________ HIV:__________

Others: ____

Ultrasonography: ____

REMARKS

Diet Ordered: ____

____

______________________________ Medication: ______________________________

____

Nursing Interventions:____

____

Health Education:____

____

____

____

Sign of Supervisor **Sign of Student**

ANTENATAL EXAMINATION

Name:________________ Age:__________ G, P, L, A ________________
Name of the Hospital:________________ Hospital Number: ________________
Date of Admission:________________ Weeks of Gestation:________________
Date of Registration:__________ LMP: __________ EDD: ________________
High-risk Pregnancy Group: Yes/No

MEDICAL HISTORY

Chronic Illness:________________
Surgery:________________
Allergy:________________
Communicable Disease: ________________

FAMILY HISTORY

Type of Family:
Nuclear:________________ Number of persons:________________
Joint:________________ Number of persons: ________________

HISTORY OF MULTIPLE BIRTHS

Number of Children:__________ Girl Child:__________ Boy Child:__________

SOCIOECONOMIC BACKGROUND

Religion:________________ Family Income:________________
Education: Husband: ________________ Wife: ________________
Occupation: Husband: ________________ Wife: ________________

MENSTRUAL HISTORY

Menarchy:__________ Duration:__________ Interval:__________ Flow:__________

MARITAL HISTORY

Age of Marriage:________________
Consanguineous: Yes/No

DIETARY PATTERN

Vegetarian:________________ Nonvegetarian: ________________
Likes:________________ Dislikes: ________________
Habits: Smoking/Drinking Alchohol/Chewing pan/Tobacco

HISTORY OF PREVIOUS PREGNANCIES

S. No.	Year	Full Term	Pre-mature	Abortion	Mode of Delivery	puerpe-rium	CHILD				
							Alive	Stillborn	Sex	Wt. at Birth	Growth and Develop

Diet Ordered: ____________________

Medications Ordered: ____________________

Treatment: ____________________

Remarks: ____________________

Nursing Intervention and Health Education:

PRENATAL VISITS

Date	Height	Weight	Urine	BP	FHR	Ht. of Fundus	Abd. Girth	Presenta-tion	Position	Treatment Remarks

GENERAL EXAMINATION

Date of Admission:________________ Diagnosis:________________

General condition: Good/Fair/Satisfactory/Poor

Heart:________ Lungs:________ Abdomen:________

Breast:________ Nipples:________

Edema Ankles:________ Hands:________

TPR:________ BP________

Digestion:________ Micturation:________

Vaginal Discharge:________

INVESTIGATION

Blood Group:________ Rh Factor:________ Hb:________ VDRL:________ HIV:________

Others:________

Ultrasonography:________

REMARKS

Diet Ordered:________

____

________ Medication:________

____

Nursing Interventions:________

____

Health Education:________

____

____

____

Sign of Supervisor **Sign of Student**

ANTENATAL EXAMINATION

Name:__________ Age: __________ G, P, L, A __________
Name of the Hospital:__________ Hospital Number: __________
Date of Admission:__________ Weeks of Gestation:__________
Date of Registration:__________ LMP: __________ EDD: __________
High-risk Pregnancy Group: Yes/No

MEDICAL HISTORY

Chronic Illness:__________
Surgery:__________
Allergy:__________
Communicable Disease: __________

FAMILY HISTORY

Type of Family:
Nuclear:__________ Number of persons:__________
Joint:__________ Number of persons: __________

HISTORY OF MULTIPLE BIRTHS

Number of Children:__________ Girl Child:__________ Boy Child:__________

SOCIOECONOMIC BACKGROUND

Religion:__________ Family Income:__________
Education: Husband: __________ Wife: __________
Occupation: Husband: __________ Wife: __________

MENSTRUAL HISTORY

Menarchy:__________ Duration:__________ Interval:__________ Flow:__________

MARITAL HISTORY

Age of Marriage:__________
Consanguineous: Yes/No

DIETARY PATTERN

Vegetarian:__________ Nonvegetarian: __________
Likes:__________ Dislikes: __________
Habits: Smoking/Drinking Alchohol/Chewing pan/Tobacco

HISTORY OF PREVIOUS PREGNANCIES

S. No.	Year	Full Term	Pre-mature	Abortion	Mode of Delivery	puerpe-rium	CHILD				
							Alive	Stillborn	Sex	Wt. at Birth	Growth and Develop

Diet Ordered:__________

Medications Ordered: __________

Treatment: __________

Remarks:__________

Nursing Intervention and Health Education:

PRENATAL VISITS

Date	Height	Weight	Urine	BP	FHR	Ht. of Fundus	Abd. Girth	Presenta-tion	Position	Treatment Remarks

GENERAL EXAMINATION

Date of Admission:__________________ Diagnosis:__________________
General condition: Good/Fair/Satisfactory/Poor
Heart: __________ Lungs:__________ Abdomen:__________
Breast:__________Nipples:__________
Edema Ankles:__________Hands:__________
TPR: __________ BP __________
Digestion: __________ Micturation: __________
Vaginal Discharge:__________

INVESTIGATION

Blood Group:__________ Rh Factor:__________ Hb:__________ VDRL:__________ HIV:__________
Others: __________
Ultrasonography: __________

REMARKS

Diet Ordered: __________
____
__________ Medication: __________
____

Nursing Interventions:__________
____

Health Education:__________
____
____
____

Sign of Supervisor **Sign of Student**

ANTENATAL EXAMINATION

Name:________________________ Age: ____________ G, P, L, A ____________________
Name of the Hospital:____________________ Hospital Number: ____________________
Date of Admission:______________________ Weeks of Gestation:__________________
Date of Registration:____________ LMP: ____________ EDD: ____________________
High-risk Pregnancy Group: Yes/No

MEDICAL HISTORY

Chronic Illness:____
Surgery:____
Allergy:____
Communicable Disease: ____

FAMILY HISTORY

Type of Family:
Nuclear:______________________________ Number of persons:____________________
Joint:______________________________ Number of persons: ____________________

HISTORY OF MULTIPLE BIRTHS

Number of Children:________________ Girl Child:______________ Boy Child:______________

SOCIOECONOMIC BACKGROUND

Religion:______________________________ Family Income:____________________
Education: Husband: ______________________________ Wife: ____________________
Occupation: Husband: ______________________________ Wife: ____________________

MENSTRUAL HISTORY

Menarchy:______________ Duration:______________ Interval:______________ Flow:__________

MARITAL HISTORY

Age of Marriage:______________________________
Consanguineous: Yes/No

DIETARY PATTERN

Vegetarian:______________________________ Nonvegetarian: ____________________
Likes:______________________________ Dislikes: ____________________
Habits: Smoking/Drinking Alchohol/Chewing pan/Tobacco

HISTORY OF PREVIOUS PREGNANCIES

S. No.	Year	Full Term	Pre-mature	Abortion	Mode of Delivery	puerpe-rium	CHILD				
							Alive	Stillborn	Sex	Wt. at Birth	Growth and Develop

Diet Ordered:____________________

Medications Ordered: ____________________

____

Treatment: ____________________

____

Remarks:____________________

Nursing Intervention and Health Education:

PRENATAL VISITS

Date	Height	Weight	Urine	BP	FHR	Ht. of Fundus	Abd. Girth	Presenta-tion	Position	Treatment Remarks

GENERAL EXAMINATION

Date of Admission:__________ Diagnosis:__________

General condition: Good/Fair/Satisfactory/Poor

Heart: __________ Lungs:__________ Abdomen:__________

Breast:__________ Nipples:__________

Edema Ankles:__________ Hands:__________

TPR: __________ BP __________

Digestion: __________ Micturation: __________

Vaginal Discharge:__________

INVESTIGATION

Blood Group:__________ Rh Factor:__________ Hb:__________ VDRL:__________ HIV:__________

Others: __________

Ultrasonography: __________

REMARKS

Diet Ordered: __________

____

__________ Medication: __________

____

Nursing Interventions:__________

____

Health Education:__________

____

____

____

Sign of Supervisor **Sign of Student**

ANTENATAL EXAMINATION

Name:__________ Age: __________ G, P, L, A __________
Name of the Hospital:__________ Hospital Number: __________
Date of Admission:__________ Weeks of Gestation:__________
Date of Registration:__________ LMP: __________ EDD: __________
High-risk Pregnancy Group: Yes/No

MEDICAL HISTORY

Chronic Illness:__________
Surgery:__________
Allergy:__________
Communicable Disease: __________

FAMILY HISTORY

Type of Family:
Nuclear:__________ Number of persons:__________
Joint:__________ Number of persons: __________

HISTORY OF MULTIPLE BIRTHS

Number of Children:__________ Girl Child:__________ Boy Child:__________

SOCIOECONOMIC BACKGROUND

Religion:__________ Family Income:__________
Education: Husband: __________ Wife: __________
Occupation: Husband: __________ Wife: __________

MENSTRUAL HISTORY

Menarchy:__________ Duration:__________ Interval:__________ Flow:__________

MARITAL HISTORY

Age of Marriage:__________
Consanguineous: Yes/No

DIETARY PATTERN

Vegetarian:__________ Nonvegetarian: __________
Likes:__________ Dislikes: __________
Habits: Smoking/Drinking Alchohol/Chewing pan/Tobacco

HISTORY OF PREVIOUS PREGNANCIES

S. No.	Year	Full Term	Pre-mature	Abortion	Mode of Delivery	puerpe-rium	CHILD				
							Alive	Stillborn	Sex	Wt. at Birth	Growth and Develop

Diet Ordered: ____________________

Medications Ordered: ____________________

____

Treatment: ____________________

____

Remarks: ____________________

Nursing Intervention and Health Education:

____

____

____

____

____

____

____

____

____

____

____

PRENATAL VISITS

Date	Height	Weight	Urine	BP	FHR	Ht. of Fundus	Abd. Girth	Presenta-tion	Position	Treatment Remarks

GENERAL EXAMINATION

Date of Admission:____________ Diagnosis:____________

General condition: Good/Fair/Satisfactory/Poor

Heart: ________ Lungs:________ Abdomen:________

Breast:____________ Nipples:____________

Edema Ankles:____________ Hands:____________

TPR: ____________ BP ____________

Digestion: ____________ Micturation: ____________

Vaginal Discharge:____________

INVESTIGATION

Blood Group:________ Rh Factor:________ Hb:________ VDRL:________ HIV:________

Others: ____________

Ultrasonography: ____________

REMARKS

Diet Ordered: ____________

____

____________ Medication: ____________

____

Nursing Interventions:____________

____

Health Education:____________

____

____

____

Sign of Supervisor **Sign of Student**

ANTENATAL EXAMINATION

Name:________________ Age: ________ G, P, L, A ________________
Name of the Hospital:________________ Hospital Number: ________________
Date of Admission:________________ Weeks of Gestation:________________
Date of Registration:__________ LMP: __________ EDD: ________________
High-risk Pregnancy Group: Yes/No

MEDICAL HISTORY

Chronic Illness:________________________________
Surgery:________________________________
Allergy:________________________________
Communicable Disease: ________________________________

FAMILY HISTORY

Type of Family:
Nuclear:________________ Number of persons:________________
Joint:________________ Number of persons: ________________

HISTORY OF MULTIPLE BIRTHS

Number of Children:__________ Girl Child:__________ Boy Child:__________

SOCIOECONOMIC BACKGROUND

Religion:________________ Family Income:________________
Education: Husband: ________________ Wife: ________________
Occupation: Husband: ________________ Wife: ________________

MENSTRUAL HISTORY

Menarchy:__________ Duration:__________ Interval:__________ Flow:__________

MARITAL HISTORY

Age of Marriage:________________
Consanguineous: Yes/No

DIETARY PATTERN

Vegetarian:________________ Nonvegetarian: ________________
Likes:________________ Dislikes: ________________
Habits: Smoking/Drinking Alchohol/Chewing pan/Tobacco

HISTORY OF PREVIOUS PREGNANCIES

S. No.	Year	Full Term	Pre-mature	Abortion	Mode of Delivery	puerpe-rium	CHILD				
							Alive	Stillborn	Sex	Wt. at Birth	Growth and Develop

Diet Ordered:__________

Medications Ordered: __________

Treatment: __________

Remarks:__________

Nursing Intervention and Health Education:

PRENATAL VISITS

Date	Height	Weight	Urine	BP	FHR	Ht. of Fundus	Abd. Girth	Presenta-tion	Position	Treatment Remarks

GENERAL EXAMINATION

Date of Admission:__________ Diagnosis:__________
General condition: Good/Fair/Satisfactory/Poor
Heart: __________ Lungs:__________ Abdomen:__________
Breast:__________ Nipples:__________
Edema Ankles:__________ Hands:__________
TPR: __________ BP __________
Digestion: __________ Micturation: __________
Vaginal Discharge:__________

INVESTIGATION

Blood Group:__________ Rh Factor:__________ Hb:__________ VDRL:__________ HIV:__________
Others: __________
Ultrasonography: __________

REMARKS

Diet Ordered: __________

__________ Medication: __________

Nursing Interventions:__________

Health Education:__________

Sign of Supervisor **Sign of Student**

ANTENATAL EXAMINATION

Name:________ Age: ________ G, P, L, A ________
Name of the Hospital:________ Hospital Number: ________
Date of Admission:________ Weeks of Gestation:________
Date of Registration:________ LMP: ________ EDD: ________
High-risk Pregnancy Group: Yes/No

MEDICAL HISTORY

Chronic Illness:________
Surgery:________
Allergy:________
Communicable Disease: ________

FAMILY HISTORY

Type of Family:
Nuclear:________ Number of persons:________
Joint:________ Number of persons: ________

HISTORY OF MULTIPLE BIRTHS

Number of Children:________ Girl Child:________ Boy Child:________

SOCIOECONOMIC BACKGROUND

Religion:________ Family Income:________
Education: Husband: ________ Wife: ________
Occupation: Husband: ________ Wife: ________

MENSTRUAL HISTORY

Menarchy:________ Duration:________ Interval:________ Flow:________

MARITAL HISTORY

Age of Marriage:________
Consanguineous: Yes/No

DIETARY PATTERN

Vegetarian:________ Nonvegetarian: ________
Likes:________ Dislikes: ________
Habits: Smoking/Drinking Alchohol/Chewing pan/Tobacco

HISTORY OF PREVIOUS PREGNANCIES

S. No.	Year	Full Term	Pre-mature	Abortion	Mode of Delivery	puerpe-rium	CHILD				
							Alive	Stillborn	Sex	Wt. at Birth	Growth and Develop

Diet Ordered:

Medications Ordered:

Treatment:

Remarks:

Nursing Intervention and Health Education:

PRENATAL VISITS

Date	Height	Weight	Urine	BP	FHR	Ht. of Fundus	Abd. Girth	Presenta-tion	Position	Treatment Remarks

GENERAL EXAMINATION

Date of Admission:____________________ Diagnosis:____________________
General condition: Good/Fair/Satisfactory/Poor
Heart: __________ Lungs:__________ Abdomen:__________
Breast:__________ Nipples:__________
Edema Ankles:__________ Hands:__________
TPR: __________ BP __________
Digestion: __________ Micturation: __________
Vaginal Discharge:____________________

INVESTIGATION

Blood Group:__________ Rh Factor:__________ Hb:__________ VDRL:__________ HIV:__________
Others: ____________________
Ultrasonography: ____________________

REMARKS

Diet Ordered: ____________________
____
__________ Medication: ____________________
____

Nursing Interventions:____________________
____

Health Education:____________________
____
____
____

Sign of Supervisor **Sign of Student**

ANTENATAL EXAMINATION

Name:________________ Age:________ G, P, L, A ________________
Name of the Hospital:________________ Hospital Number: ________________
Date of Admission:________________ Weeks of Gestation:________________
Date of Registration:__________ LMP: __________ EDD: ________________
High-risk Pregnancy Group: Yes/No

MEDICAL HISTORY

Chronic Illness:________________
Surgery:________________
Allergy:________________
Communicable Disease: ________________

FAMILY HISTORY

Type of Family:
Nuclear:________________ Number of persons:________________
Joint:________________ Number of persons: ________________

HISTORY OF MULTIPLE BIRTHS

Number of Children:__________ Girl Child:__________ Boy Child:__________

SOCIOECONOMIC BACKGROUND

Religion:________________ Family Income:________________
Education: Husband: ________________ Wife: ________________
Occupation: Husband: ________________ Wife: ________________

MENSTRUAL HISTORY

Menarchy:__________ Duration:__________ Interval:__________ Flow:__________

MARITAL HISTORY

Age of Marriage:________________
Consanguineous: Yes/No

DIETARY PATTERN

Vegetarian:________________ Nonvegetarian: ________________
Likes:________________ Dislikes: ________________
Habits: Smoking/Drinking Alchohol/Chewing pan/Tobacco

HISTORY OF PREVIOUS PREGNANCIES

S. No.	Year	Full Term	Pre-mature	Abortion	Mode of Delivery	puerpe-rium	CHILD				
							Alive	Stillborn	Sex	Wt. at Birth	Growth and Develop

Diet Ordered:__________

Medications Ordered: __________

Treatment: __________

Remarks:__________

Nursing Intervention and Health Education:

PRENATAL VISITS

Date	Height	Weight	Urine	BP	FHR	Ht. of Fundus	Abd. Girth	Presenta-tion	Position	Treatment Remarks

GENERAL EXAMINATION

Date of Admission:________________________ Diagnosis:________________________

General condition: Good/Fair/Satisfactory/Poor

Heart: ____________ Lungs:________________ Abdomen:________________

Breast:________________ Nipples:________________________

Edema Ankles:________________________ Hands:________________________

TPR: ________________________ BP ________________________

Digestion: ________________________ Micturation: ________________________

Vaginal Discharge:____

INVESTIGATION

Blood Group:__________ Rh Factor:__________ Hb:__________ VDRL:__________ HIV:__________

Others: ____

Ultrasonography: ____

REMARKS

Diet Ordered: ____

____

________________________ Medication: ________________________

____

Nursing Interventions:____

____

Health Education:____

____

____

____

Sign of Supervisor **Sign of Student**

ANTENATAL EXAMINATION

Name:_______________ Age: _______________ G, P, L, A _______________
Name of the Hospital:_______________ Hospital Number: _______________
Date of Admission:_______________ Weeks of Gestation:_______________
Date of Registration:_______________ LMP: _______________ EDD: _______________
High-risk Pregnancy Group: Yes/No

MEDICAL HISTORY

Chronic Illness:_______________
Surgery:_______________
Allergy:_______________
Communicable Disease: _______________

FAMILY HISTORY

Type of Family:
Nuclear:_______________ Number of persons:_______________
Joint:_______________ Number of persons: _______________

HISTORY OF MULTIPLE BIRTHS

Number of Children:_______________ Girl Child:_______________ Boy Child:_______________

SOCIOECONOMIC BACKGROUND

Religion:_______________ Family Income:_______________
Education: Husband: _______________ Wife: _______________
Occupation: Husband: _______________ Wife: _______________

MENSTRUAL HISTORY

Menarchy:_______________ Duration:_______________ Interval:_______________ Flow:_______________

MARITAL HISTORY

Age of Marriage:_______________
Consanguineous: Yes/No

DIETARY PATTERN

Vegetarian:_______________ Nonvegetarian: _______________
Likes:_______________ Dislikes: _______________
Habits: Smoking/Drinking Alchohol/Chewing pan/Tobacco

HISTORY OF PREVIOUS PREGNANCIES

S. No.	Year	Full Term	Pre-mature	Abortion	Mode of Delivery	puerpe-rium	CHILD				
							Alive	Stillborn	Sex	Wt. at Birth	Growth and Develop

Diet Ordered: ___

Medications Ordered: ___

Treatment: ___

Remarks: ___

Nursing Intervention and Health Education:

PRENATAL VISITS

Date	Height	Weight	Urine	BP	FHR	Ht. of Fundus	Abd. Girth	Presenta-tion	Position	Treatment Remarks

GENERAL EXAMINATION

Date of Admission:____________________ Diagnosis:____________________

General condition: Good/Fair/Satisfactory/Poor

Heart: __________ Lungs:__________ Abdomen:__________

Breast:__________Nipples:____________________

Edema Ankles:____________________Hands:____________________

TPR: ____________________ BP ____________________

Digestion: ____________________ Micturation: ____________________

Vaginal Discharge:____

INVESTIGATION

Blood Group:__________ Rh Factor:__________ Hb:__________ VDRL:__________ HIV:__________

Others: ____

Ultrasonography: ____

REMARKS

Diet Ordered: ____

____

____________________ Medication: ____________________

____

Nursing Interventions:____

____

Health Education:____

____

____

____

Sign of Supervisor **Sign of Student**

ANTENATAL EXAMINATION

Name:________________ Age: ________ G, P, L, A ________________
Name of the Hospital:________________ Hospital Number: ________________
Date of Admission:________________ Weeks of Gestation:________________
Date of Registration:__________ LMP: __________ EDD: ________________
High-risk Pregnancy Group: Yes/No

MEDICAL HISTORY

Chronic Illness:________________
Surgery:________________
Allergy:________________
Communicable Disease: ________________

FAMILY HISTORY

Type of Family:
Nuclear:________________ Number of persons:________________
Joint:________________ Number of persons: ________________

HISTORY OF MULTIPLE BIRTHS

Number of Children:__________ Girl Child:__________ Boy Child:__________

SOCIOECONOMIC BACKGROUND

Religion:________________ Family Income:________________
Education: Husband: ________________ Wife: ________________
Occupation: Husband: ________________ Wife: ________________

MENSTRUAL HISTORY

Menarchy:__________ Duration:__________ Interval:__________ Flow:__________

MARITAL HISTORY

Age of Marriage:________________
Consanguineous: Yes/No

DIETARY PATTERN

Vegetarian:________________ Nonvegetarian: ________________
Likes:________________ Dislikes: ________________
Habits: Smoking/Drinking Alchohol/Chewing pan/Tobacco

HISTORY OF PREVIOUS PREGNANCIES

S. No.	Year	Full Term	Pre-mature	Abortion	Mode of Delivery	puerpe-rium	CHILD				
							Alive	Stillborn	Sex	Wt. at Birth	Growth and Develop

Diet Ordered:____________________

Medications Ordered: ____________________

Treatment: ____________________

Remarks:____________________

Nursing Intervention and Health Education:

PRENATAL VISITS

Date	Height	Weight	Urine	BP	FHR	Ht. of Fundus	Abd. Girth	Presenta-tion	Position	Treatment Remarks

GENERAL EXAMINATION

Date of Admission:____ Diagnosis:________________________________

General condition: Good/Fair/Satisfactory/Poor

Heart: __________________ Lungs:__________________________ Abdomen:______________________________

Breast:______________________________Nipples:____

Edema Ankles:_______________________________________Hands:____________________________________

TPR: ____ BP ____________________________________

Digestion: _____________________________________ Micturation: ______________________________________

Vaginal Discharge:____

INVESTIGATION

Blood Group:________________ Rh Factor:____________ Hb:____________ VDRL:_____________ HIV:______________

Others: ____

Ultrasonography: ____

REMARKS

Diet Ordered: ____

____

_________________________________ Medication: ____

____

Nursing Interventions:____

____

Health Education:____

____

____

____

Sign of Supervisor **Sign of Student**

ANTENATAL EXAMINATION

Name:__________ Age: __________ G, P, L, A __________
Name of the Hospital:__________ Hospital Number: __________
Date of Admission:__________ Weeks of Gestation:__________
Date of Registration:__________ LMP: __________ EDD: __________
High-risk Pregnancy Group: Yes/No

MEDICAL HISTORY

Chronic Illness:__________
Surgery:__________
Allergy:__________
Communicable Disease: __________

FAMILY HISTORY

Type of Family:
Nuclear:__________ Number of persons:__________
Joint:__________ Number of persons: __________

HISTORY OF MULTIPLE BIRTHS

Number of Children:__________ Girl Child:__________ Boy Child:__________

SOCIOECONOMIC BACKGROUND

Religion:__________ Family Income:__________
Education: Husband: __________ Wife: __________
Occupation: Husband: __________ Wife: __________

MENSTRUAL HISTORY

Menarchy:__________ Duration:__________ Interval:__________ Flow:__________

MARITAL HISTORY

Age of Marriage:__________
Consanguineous: Yes/No

DIETARY PATTERN

Vegetarian:__________ Nonvegetarian: __________
Likes:__________ Dislikes: __________
Habits: Smoking/Drinking Alchohol/Chewing pan/Tobacco

HISTORY OF PREVIOUS PREGNANCIES

S. No.	Year	Full Term	Pre-mature	Abortion	Mode of Delivery	puerpe-rium	CHILD				
							Alive	Stillborn	Sex	Wt. at Birth	Growth and Develop

Diet Ordered: ____________________

Medications Ordered: ____________________

Treatment: ____________________

Remarks: ____________________

Nursing Intervention and Health Education:

PRENATAL VISITS

Date	Height	Weight	Urine	BP	FHR	Ht. of Fundus	Abd. Girth	Presenta-tion	Position	Treatment Remarks

GENERAL EXAMINATION

Date of Admission:______________________ Diagnosis:______________________
General condition: Good/Fair/Satisfactory/Poor
Heart: ______________ Lungs:______________ Abdomen:______________
Breast:______________________ Nipples:______________________
Edema Ankles:______________________ Hands:______________________
TPR: ______________________ BP ______________________
Digestion: ______________________ Micturation: ______________________
Vaginal Discharge:______________________

INVESTIGATION

Blood Group:__________ Rh Factor:__________ Hb:__________ VDRL:__________ HIV:__________
Others: ______________________
Ultrasonography: ______________________

REMARKS

Diet Ordered: ______________________
____
______________________ Medication: ______________________
____

Nursing Interventions:______________________
____

Health Education:______________________
____
____
____

Sign of Supervisor **Sign of Student**

INTRANATAL EXAMINATION

INTRANATAL CASE STUDY

Name:__________ Age: ______ G, P, L, A __________
Name of the Hospital:__________ Hospital Number: __________
Date of Admission:__________

ANTENATAL RECORD

Date of Booking:______ LMP:______ EDD:______ Gestation at 1st Visit:______

MEDICAL HISTORY

Chronic Illness:__________
Surgery:__________
Allergy:__________
Communicable Disease:__________

FAMILY HISTORY

Type of Family:
Nuclear: __________ Number of Persons: __________
Joint: __________ Number of Persons: __________

DISEASES: Chronic Illness

Hypertension:______ Diabetes:______ Genetic Diseases:______ Psychiatric Disorders:______
Others : __________

HISTORY OF MULTIPLE BIRTHS

Number of Children :______ Girl Child:______ Boy Child______

SOCIOECONOMIC BACKGROUND

Religion:__________ Family Income:__________
Education: Husband: __________ Wife: __________
Occupation: Husband: __________ Wife: __________

MENSTRUAL HISTORY

Menarchy:______ Duration:______ Interval:______ Flow:______

MARITAL HISTORY

Age of Marriage:__________
Consanguineous: Yes/No

DIETARY PATTERN

Vegetarian: __________ Nonvegetarian: __________
Likes:__________ Dislikes:__________
Habits: Smoking/Drinking Alchohol/Chewing Pan/Tobacco

PAST OBSTETRICAL HISTORY

S.No	Year	Full Term	Abortion	Type of Delivery	Sex of Baby	Alive	Stillbirth	Weight	Remarks

PRESENT PREGNANCY

Admission Notes:

Admission on:__________ at:__________ Contractions Commenced:__________ at:__________
Period of Gestation:__________ Membranes: Intact:__________ Ruptured on:__________
Height of Fundus:__________ Contractions__________
Presentation:__________ Position:__________
Engaged/Nonengaged:__________ FHR:__________
Bladder:__________ Bowel:__________
BP:__________ TPR:__________
Special Observations:__________

PRENATAL VISITS

Date of Booking	Weight	Height	Urine		BP	FHR	Weeks of Gestation	Height of Fundus	Position	Treatment
			Protein	Glucose						

EXAMINATION AND INVESTIGATIONS

Blood Group:________ Rh Factor:________ Hb:________ VDRL:________ HIV:________ Others:________
Heart________ Lungs________ Breast________ Abdomen________ Perineum________

DELIVERY RECORD

Onset of True Labour: Date:__________ Time:__________
Time of Full Dilatation: Date:__________ Time:__________
Membranes Ruptured at:__________ Spontaneous/Artificial:__________ PROM:__________

THE SIMPLIFIED PARTOGRAPH

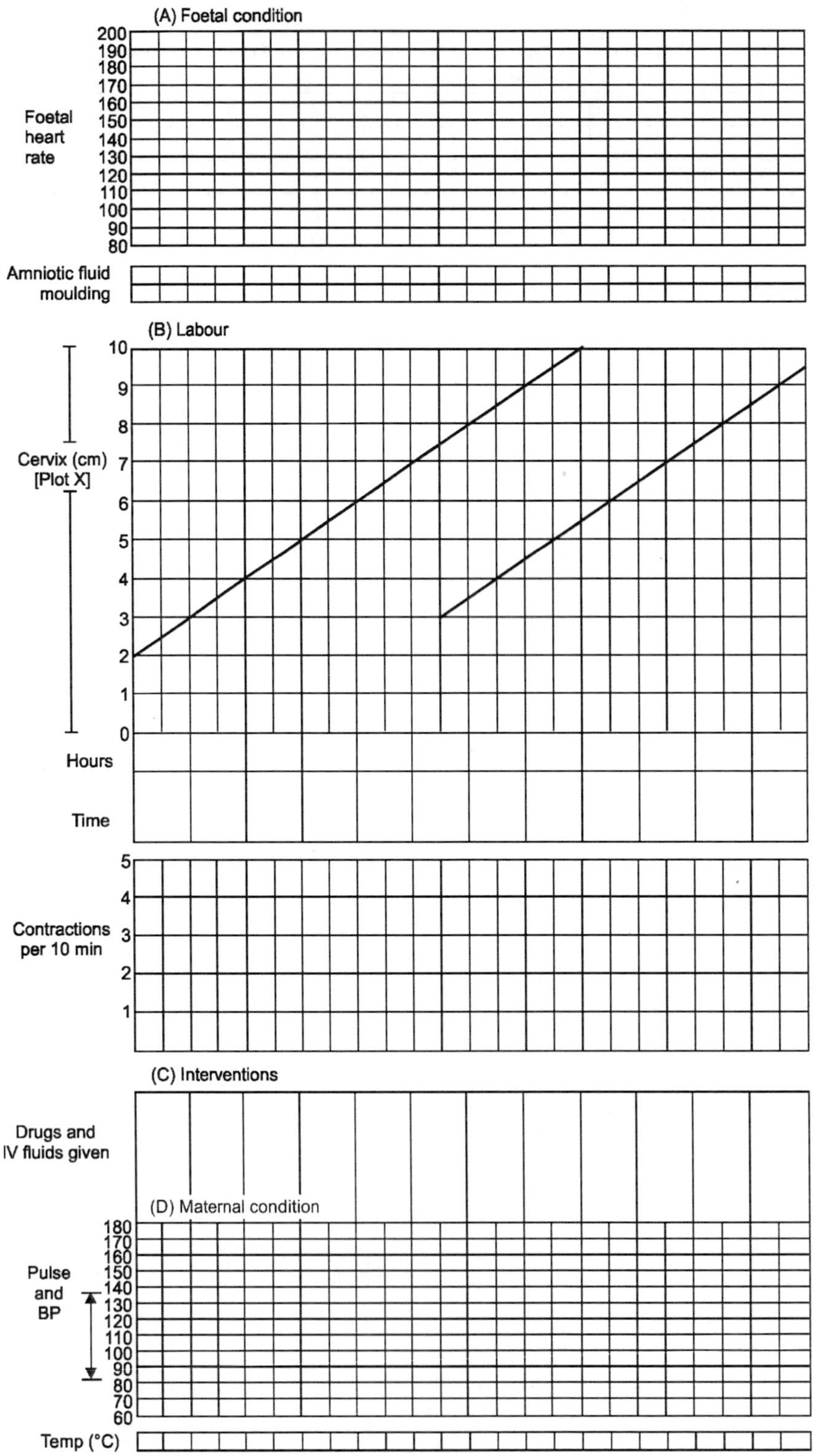

a. Delivery of Baby

Baby Born at:______________ AM/PM, Male/Female:______________________ Mode of Delivery: __________________
Condition of Baby: Active/ Nonactive/Asphyxiated ____

b. Delivery of Placenta and Membranes

Delivery at:____________________________________ AM/PM
Spontaneously/Manually Removed ____
Typeofplacenta____
PlacentaandMembranes: Complete/ Incomplete____
Weight_______________Cord Length_______________________Any Abnormality____________________

c. Blood Loss (Approximate Total Amount)

Before Delivery of the Placenta___________________________ ml
During Delivery of the Placenta___________________________ml
After Delivery of the Placenta_____________________________ml
Total Amount__________________________ ml

d. Perineum

Intact__________________Episiotomy____________________Laceration__________________Repair_______________

e. Medicationsgiven____

f. Length of Labour

Duration of Labour

Progress of Labour	Date	Time	Total...... Hrs..... Min.....
Contraction Started			...... Hrs..... Min.....
Full Dilatation			
Delivery of Baby			...... Hrs..... Min.....
Delivery of Placenta			...... Hrs..... Min.....
Total Time Taken for Labour			

Condition of the Mother following Delivery

Pulse_______________BP__________________ Height of Uterus_______________ Vaginal Bleeding______________________
Breastfeeding Initiated at ____

Sign of Supervisor **Sign of Student**

INTRANATAL CASE STUDY

Name:__________ Age: __________ G, P, L, A __________
Name of the Hospital:__________ Hospital Number: __________
Date of Admission:__________

ANTENATAL RECORD

Date of Booking:__________ LMP:__________ EDD:__________ Gestation at 1st Visit:__________

MEDICAL HISTORY

Chronic Illness:__________
Surgery:__________
Allergy:__________
Communicable Disease:__________

FAMILY HISTORY

Type of Family:
Nuclear: __________ Number of Persons: __________
Joint: __________ Number of Persons: __________

DISEASES: Chronic Illness

Hypertension:__________ Diabetes:__________ Genetic Diseases:__________ Psychiatric Disorders:__________
Others : __________

HISTORY OF MULTIPLE BIRTHS

Number of Children :__________ Girl Child:__________ Boy Child__________

SOCIOECONOMIC BACKGROUND

Religion:__________ Family Income:__________
Education: Husband: __________ Wife: __________
Occupation: Husband: __________ Wife: __________

MENSTRUAL HISTORY

Menarchy:__________ Duration:__________ Interval:__________ Flow:__________

MARITAL HISTORY

Age of Marriage:__________
Consanguineous: Yes/No

DIETARY PATTERN

Vegetarian: __________ Nonvegetarian: __________
Likes:__________ Dislikes:__________
Habits: Smoking/Drinking Alchohol/Chewing Pan/Tobacco

PAST OBSTETRICAL HISTORY

S.No	Year	Full Term	Abortion	Type of Delivery	Sex of Baby	Alive	Stillbirth	Weight	Remarks

PRESENT PREGNANCY

Admission Notes:

Admission on:____________ at: ____________ Contractions Commenced:____________ at:____________

Period of Gestation:____________ Membranes: Intact:____________ Ruptured on:____________

Height of Fundus: ____________ Contractions ____________

Presentation:____________ Position:____________

Engaged/Nonengaged: ____________ FHR: ____________

Bladder :____________ Bowel:____________

BP:____________ TPR: ____________

Special Observations: ____________

PRENATAL VISITS

Date of Booking	Weight	Height	Urine		BP	FHR	Weeks of Gestation	Height of Fundus	Position	Treatment
			Protein	Glucose						

EXAMINATION AND INVESTIGATIONS

Blood Group:________ Rh Factor:________ Hb:________ VDRL:________ HIV:________Others:________

Heart________ Lungs________ Breast________ Abdomen________ Perineum________

DELIVERY RECORD

Onset of True Labour: Date:____________ Time:____________

Time of Full Dilatation: Date:____________ Time:____________

Membranes Ruptured at:____________ Spontaneous/Artificial: ____________ PROM:____________

THE SIMPLIFIED PARTOGRAPH

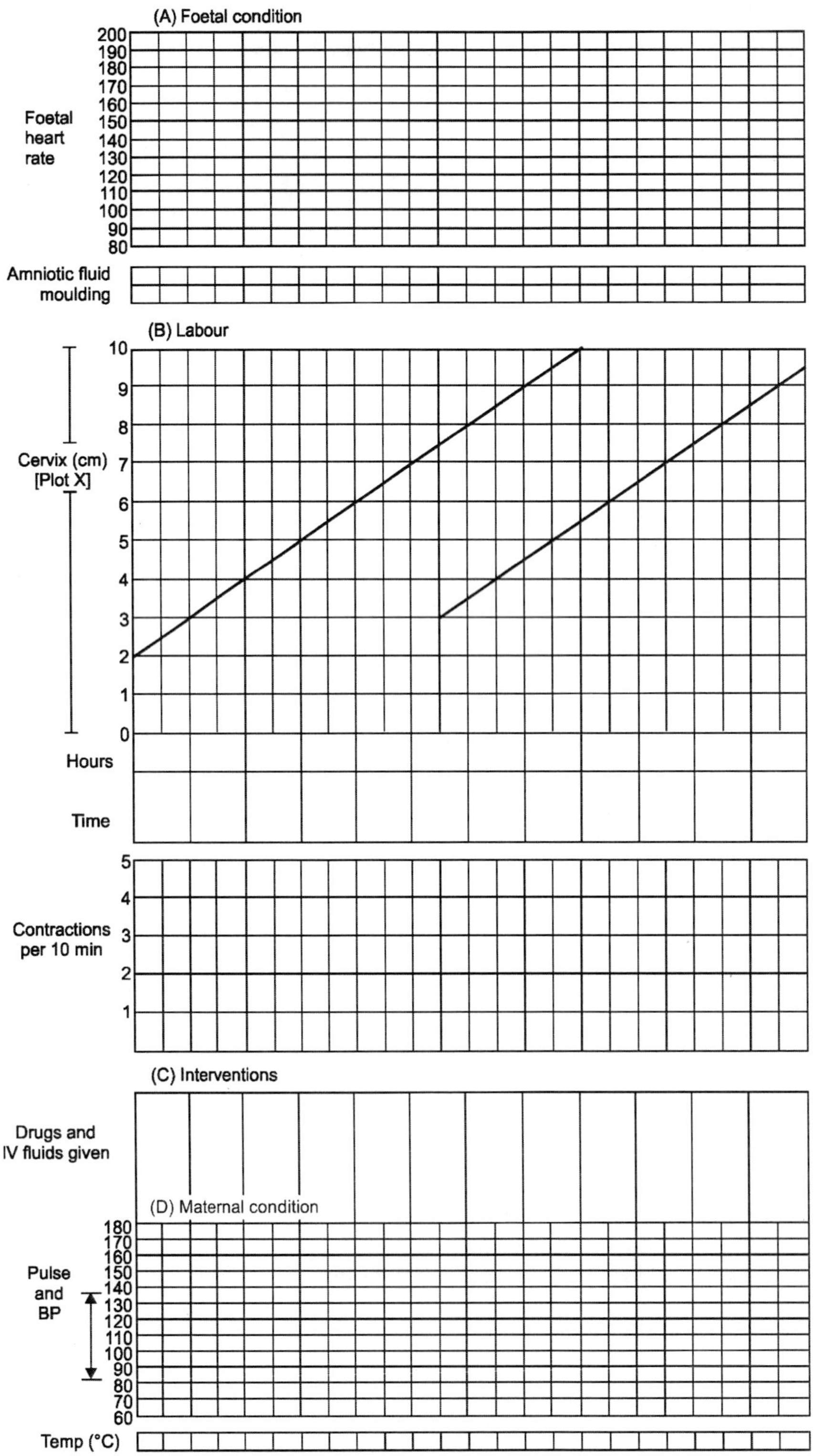

a. Delivery of Baby

Baby Born at:_____________ AM/PM, Male/Female:____________________ Mode of Delivery: _________________
Condition of Baby: Active/ Nonactive/Asphyxiated ____

b. Delivery of Placenta and Membranes

Delivery at:________________________________ AM/PM
Spontaneously/Manually Removed ____
Typeofplacenta____
PlacentaandMembranes: Complete/Incomplete____
Weight_____________CordLength____________________AnyAbnormality___________________________

c. Blood Loss (Approximate Total Amount)

Before Delivery of the Placenta________________________ ml
During Delivery of the Placenta________________________ml
After Delivery of the Placenta_________________________ml
Total Amount______________________ ml

d. Perineum

Intact________________Episiotomy_________________Laceration________________Repair_____________

e. Medicationsgiven____

f. Length of Labour

Duration of Labour

Progress of Labour	Date	Time	Total...... Hrs..... Min.....
Contraction Started			...... Hrs..... Min.....
Full Dilatation			
Delivery of Baby			...... Hrs..... Min.....
Delivery of Placenta			...... Hrs..... Min.....
Total Time Taken for Labour			

Condition of the Mother following Delivery

Pulse_____________BP________________ Height of Uterus_____________ Vaginal Bleeding____________________
Breastfeeding Initiated at ____________________________________

Sign of Supervisor **Sign of Student**

INTRANATAL CASE STUDY

Name:________ Age: ________ G, P, L, A ________
Name of the Hospital:________ Hospital Number: ________
Date of Admission:________

ANTENATAL RECORD

Date of Booking:________ LMP:________ EDD:________ Gestation at 1st Visit:________

MEDICAL HISTORY

Chronic Illness:________
Surgery:________
Allergy:________
Communicable Disease:________

FAMILY HISTORY

Type of Family:
Nuclear: ________ Number of Persons: ________
Joint: ________ Number of Persons: ________

DISEASES: Chronic Illness

Hypertension:________ Diabetes:________ Genetic Diseases:________ Psychiatric Disorders:________
Others : ________

HISTORY OF MULTIPLE BIRTHS

Number of Children :________ Girl Child:________ Boy Child________

SOCIOECONOMIC BACKGROUND

Religion:________ Family Income:________
Education: Husband: ________ Wife: ________
Occupation: Husband: ________ Wife: ________

MENSTRUAL HISTORY

Menarchy:________ Duration:________ Interval:________ Flow:________

MARITAL HISTORY

Age of Marriage:________
Consanguineous: Yes/No

DIETARY PATTERN

Vegetarian: ________ Nonvegetarian: ________
Likes:________ Dislikes:________
Habits: Smoking/Drinking Alchohol/Chewing Pan/Tobacco

PAST OBSTETRICAL HISTORY

S.No	Year	Full Term	Abortion	Type of Delivery	Sex of Baby	Alive	Stillbirth	Weight	Remarks

PRESENT PREGNANCY

Admission Notes:

Admission on:____________ at: _____________ Contractions Commenced:_______________ at:____________________

Period of Gestation:_____________________ Membranes: Intact:____________________ Ruptured on:_________________

Height of Fundus: ______________________________ Contractions ____________________________________

Presentation:_________________________________ Position:_______________________________________

Engaged/Nonengaged: ________________________________ FHR: ___________________________________

Bladder :____ Bowel:______________________________

BP:____ TPR: ___________________________________

Special Observations: ____

PRENATAL VISITS

Date of Booking	Weight	Height	Urine		BP	FHR	Weeks of Gestation	Height of Fundus	Position	Treatment
			Protein	Glucose						

EXAMINATION AND INVESTIGATIONS

Blood Group:________ Rh Factor:_________ Hb:__________ VDRL:__________ HIV:__________Others:________________

Heart_________ Lungs____________ Breast_____________ Abdomen________________ Perineum__________________

DELIVERY RECORD

Onset of True Labour: Date:________________________ Time:_______________________

Time of Full Dilatation: Date:______________________ Time:_______________________

Membranes Ruptured at:_____________________ Spontaneous/Artificial: ______________ PROM:__________________

THE SIMPLIFIED PARTOGRAPH

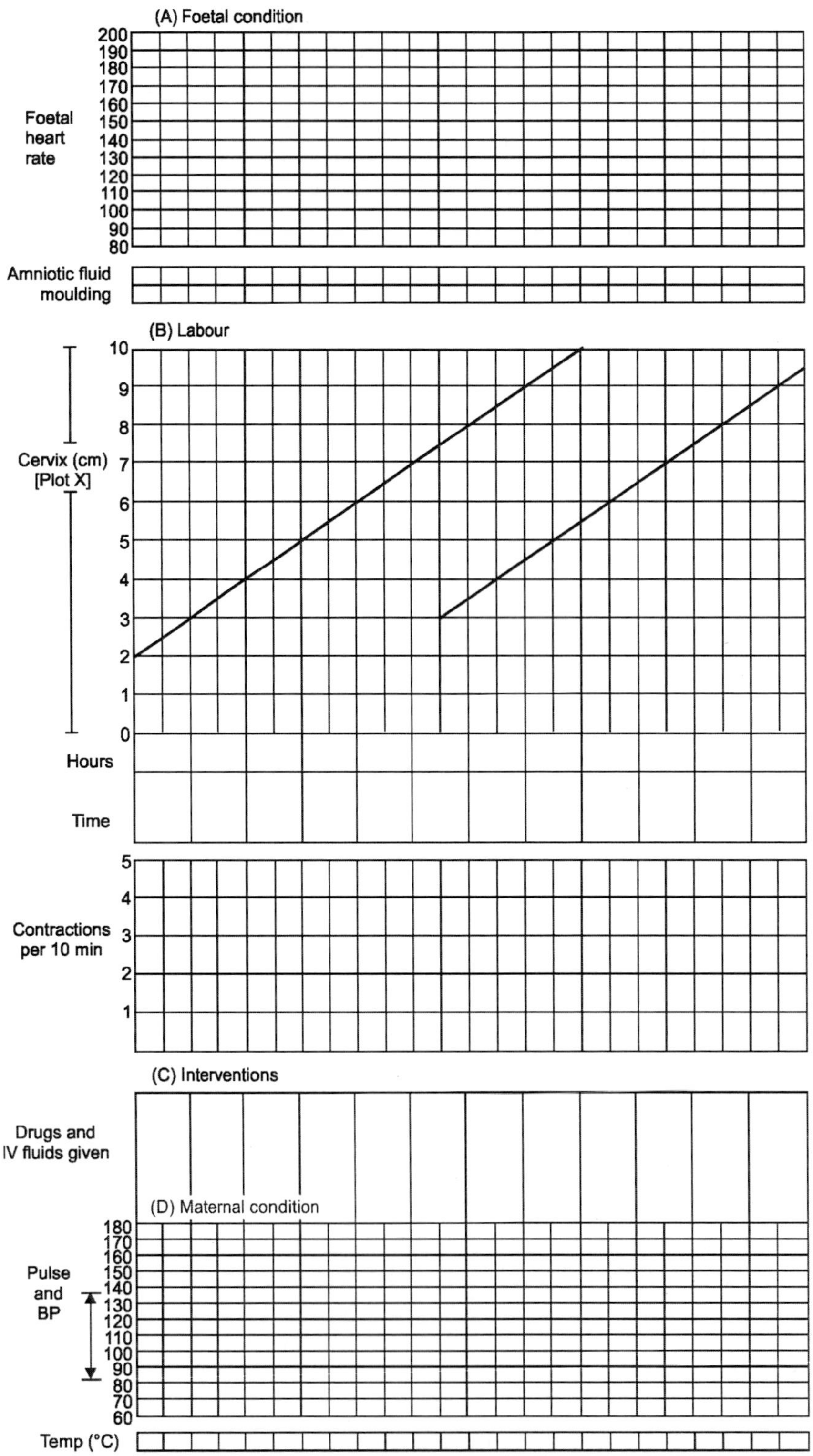

a. Delivery of Baby

Baby Born at:______________ AM/PM, Male/Female:____________________ Mode of Delivery: __________________
Condition of Baby: Active/ Nonactive/Asphyxiated ____

b. Delivery of Placenta and Membranes

Delivery at:__________________________________ AM/PM
Spontaneously/Manually Removed ____
Typeofplacenta____
PlacentaandMembranes: Complete/ Incomplete____
Weight______________Cord Length______________________Any Abnormality_________________________

c. Blood Loss (Approximate Total Amount)

Before Delivery of the Placenta_________________________ ml
During Delivery of the Placenta_________________________ml
After Delivery of the Placenta___________________________ml
Total Amount________________________ ml

d. Perineum

Intact__________________Episiotomy____________________Laceration__________________Repair_______________

e. Medicationsgiven____

f. Length of Labour

Duration of Labour

Progress of Labour	Date	Time	Total...... Hrs..... Min.....
Contraction Started			...... Hrs..... Min.....
Full Dilatation			
Delivery of Baby			...... Hrs..... Min.....
Delivery of Placenta			...... Hrs..... Min.....
Total Time Taken for Labour			

Condition of the Mother following Delivery

Pulse_______________BP__________________ Height of Uterus_______________ Vaginal Bleeding______________________
Breastfeeding Initiated at ____

Sign of Supervisor **Sign of Student**

INTRANATAL CASE STUDY

Name:____________________ Age: __________ G, P, L, A ____________________
Name of the Hospital:____________________ Hospital Number: ____________________
Date of Admission:____________________

ANTENATAL RECORD

Date of Booking:__________ LMP:__________ EDD:__________ Gestation at 1st Visit:__________

MEDICAL HISTORY

Chronic Illness:____________________
Surgery:____________________
Allergy:____________________
Communicable Disease:____________________

FAMILY HISTORY

Type of Family:
Nuclear: ____________________ Number of Persons: ____________________
Joint: ____________________ Number of Persons: ____________________

DISEASES: Chronic Illness

Hypertension:__________ Diabetes:__________ Genetic Diseases:__________ Psychiatric Disorders:__________
Others : ____________________

HISTORY OF MULTIPLE BIRTHS

Number of Children :__________ Girl Child:__________ Boy Child__________

SOCIOECONOMIC BACKGROUND

Religion:____________________ Family Income:____________________
Education: Husband: ____________________ Wife: ____________________
Occupation: Husband: ____________________ Wife: ____________________

MENSTRUAL HISTORY

Menarchy:__________ Duration:__________ Interval:__________ Flow:__________

MARITAL HISTORY

Age of Marriage:____________________
Consanguineous: Yes/No

DIETARY PATTERN

Vegetarian: ____________________ Nonvegetarian: ____________________
Likes:____________________ Dislikes:____________________
Habits: Smoking/Drinking Alchohol/Chewing Pan/Tobacco

PAST OBSTETRICAL HISTORY

S.No	Year	Full Term	Abortion	Type of Delivery	Sex of Baby	Alive	Stillbirth	Weight	Remarks

PRESENT PREGNANCY

Admission Notes:

Admission on:____________ at: _____________ Contractions Commenced:________________ at:____________________

Period of Gestation:_____________________ Membranes: Intact:____________________ Ruptured on:________________

Height of Fundus: _______________________________ Contractions ____________________________________

Presentation:_____________________________________ Position:____________________________________

Engaged/Nonengaged: ___________________________________ FHR: _____________________________________

Bladder :____ Bowel:______________________________

BP:____ TPR: ____________________________________

Special Observations: ____

PRENATAL VISITS

Date of Booking	Weight	Height	Urine		BP	FHR	Weeks of Gestation	Height of Fundus	Position	Treatment
			Protein	Glucose						

EXAMINATION AND INVESTIGATIONS

Blood Group:________ Rh Factor:_________ Hb:__________ VDRL:__________ HIV:__________Others:_______________

Heart_________ Lungs____________ Breast_____________ Abdomen________________ Perineum__________________

DELIVERY RECORD

Onset of True Labour: Date:_______________________ Time:_______________________

Time of Full Dilatation: Date:______________________ Time:_______________________

Membranes Ruptured at:______________________ Spontaneous/Artificial: ______________ PROM:__________________

THE SIMPLIFIED PARTOGRAPH

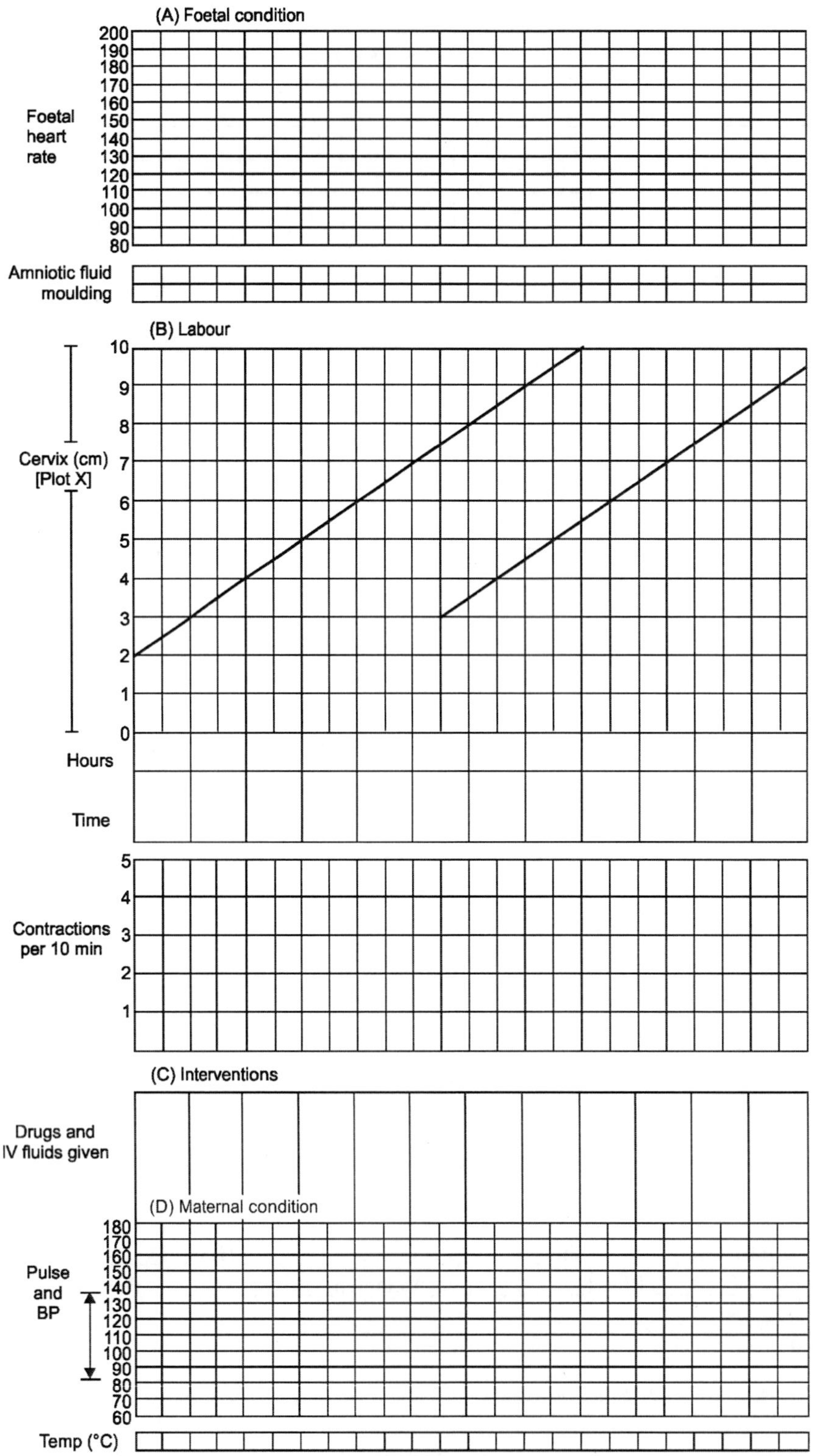

a. Delivery of Baby

Baby Born at:______________ AM/PM, Male/Female:______________________ Mode of Delivery: __________________
Condition of Baby: Active/ Nonactive/Asphyxiated ____

b. Delivery of Placenta and Membranes

Delivery at:___________________________________ AM/PM
Spontaneously/Manually Removed ____
Typeofplacenta____
PlacentaandMembranes: Complete/ Incomplete____
Weight_______________Cord Length_______________________Any Abnormality__________________________

c. Blood Loss (Approximate Total Amount)

Before Delivery of the Placenta__________________________ ml
During Delivery of the Placenta__________________________ml
After Delivery of the Placenta____________________________ml
Total Amount________________________ ml

d. Perineum

Intact___________________Episiotomy____________________Laceration__________________Repair_______________

e. Medicationsgiven____

f. Length of Labour

Duration of Labour

Progress of Labour	Date	Time	Total...... Hrs..... Min.....
Contraction Started			...... Hrs..... Min.....
Full Dilatation			
Delivery of Baby			...... Hrs..... Min.....
Delivery of Placenta			...... Hrs..... Min.....
Total Time Taken for Labour			

Condition of the Mother following Delivery

Pulse_______________BP__________________ Height of Uterus______________ Vaginal Bleeding______________________
Breastfeeding Initiated at ____

Sign of Supervisor **Sign of Student**

INTRANATAL CASE STUDY

Name:__________ Age: __________ G, P, L, A __________
Name of the Hospital:__________ Hospital Number: __________
Date of Admission:__________

ANTENATAL RECORD

Date of Booking:__________ LMP:__________ EDD:__________ Gestation at 1st Visit:__________

MEDICAL HISTORY

Chronic Illness:__________
Surgery:__________
Allergy:__________
Communicable Disease:__________

FAMILY HISTORY

Type of Family:
Nuclear: __________ Number of Persons: __________
Joint: __________ Number of Persons: __________

DISEASES: Chronic Illness

Hypertension:__________ Diabetes:__________ Genetic Diseases:__________ Psychiatric Disorders:__________
Others : __________

HISTORY OF MULTIPLE BIRTHS

Number of Children :__________ Girl Child:__________ Boy Child__________

SOCIOECONOMIC BACKGROUND

Religion:__________ Family Income:__________
Education: Husband: __________ Wife: __________
Occupation: Husband: __________ Wife: __________

MENSTRUAL HISTORY

Menarchy:__________ Duration:__________ Interval:__________ Flow:__________

MARITAL HISTORY

Age of Marriage:__________
Consanguineous: Yes/No

DIETARY PATTERN

Vegetarian: __________ Nonvegetarian: __________
Likes:__________ Dislikes:__________
Habits: Smoking/Drinking Alchohol/Chewing Pan/Tobacco

PAST OBSTETRICAL HISTORY

S.No	Year	Full Term	Abortion	Type of Delivery	Sex of Baby	Alive	Stillbirth	Weight	Remarks

PRESENT PREGNANCY

Admission Notes:

Admission on:____________ at:_____________ Contractions Commenced:______________ at:____________________

Period of Gestation:______________________ Membranes: Intact:____________________ Ruptured on:______________

Height of Fundus: ________________________________ Contractions ______________________________________

Presentation:______________________________________ Position:____

Engaged/Nonengaged: ____________________________________ FHR: _____________________________________

Bladder :____ Bowel:________________________________

BP:____ TPR: ____

Special Observations: ____

PRENATAL VISITS

Date of Booking	Weight	Height	Urine		BP	FHR	Weeks of Gestation	Height of Fundus	Position	Treatment
			Protein	Glucose						

EXAMINATION AND INVESTIGATIONS

Blood Group:________ Rh Factor:_________ Hb:__________ VDRL:__________ HIV:__________Others:________________

Heart_________ Lungs____________ Breast_____________ Abdomen________________ Perineum__________________

DELIVERY RECORD

Onset of True Labour: Date:________________________ Time:________________________

Time of Full Dilatation: Date:_______________________ Time:________________________

Membranes Ruptured at:_______________________ Spontaneous/Artificial: ______________ PROM:____________________

THE SIMPLIFIED PARTOGRAPH

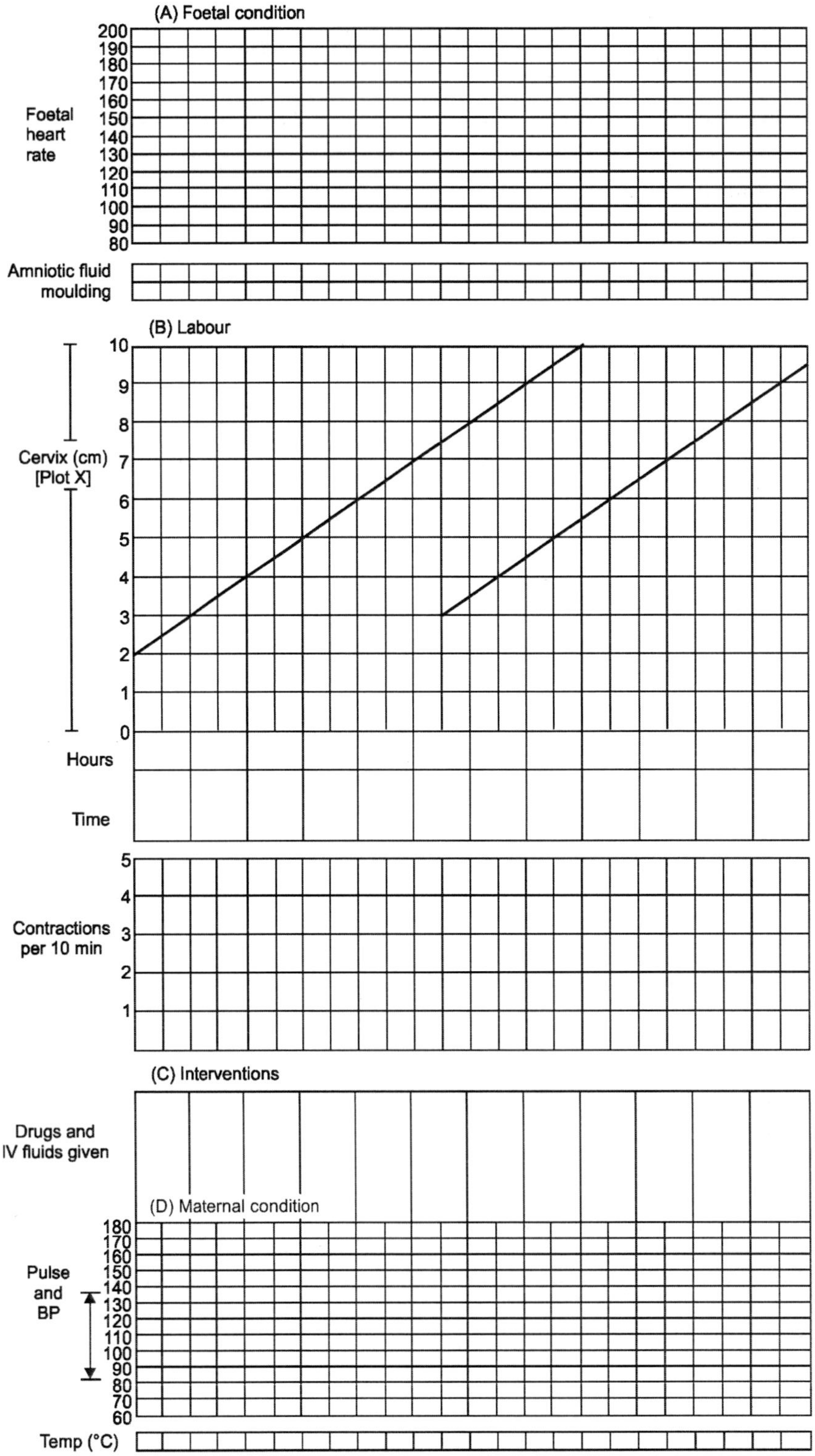

a. Delivery of Baby

Baby Born at:______________ AM/PM, Male/Female:____________________ Mode of Delivery: __________________
Condition of Baby: Active/ Nonactive/Asphyxiated ____

b. Delivery of Placenta and Membranes

Delivery at:___________________________________ AM/PM
Spontaneously/Manually Removed ____
Typeofplacenta____
PlacentaandMembranes: Complete/Incomplete____
Weight______________Cord Length______________________Any Abnormality___________________________

c. Blood Loss (Approximate Total Amount)

Before Delivery of the Placenta_________________________ ml
During Delivery of the Placenta_________________________ml
After Delivery of the Placenta___________________________ml
Total Amount________________________ ml

d. Perineum

Intact__________________Episiotomy___________________Laceration__________________Repair_______________

e. Medicationsgiven____

f. Length of Labour

Duration of Labour

Progress of Labour	Date	Time	Total...... Hrs..... Min.....
Contraction Started			...... Hrs..... Min.....
Full Dilatation			
Delivery of Baby			...... Hrs..... Min.....
Delivery of Placenta			...... Hrs..... Min.....
Total Time Taken for Labour			

Condition of the Mother following Delivery

Pulse______________BP_________________ Height of Uterus______________ Vaginal Bleeding______________________
Breastfeeding Initiated at ____

Sign of Supervisor **Sign of Student**

INTRANATAL CASE STUDY

Name:_______________ Age: _______ G, P, L, A _______________
Name of the Hospital:_______________ Hospital Number: _______________
Date of Admission:_______________

ANTENATAL RECORD

Date of Booking:__________ LMP:________ EDD:________ Gestation at 1st Visit:__________

MEDICAL HISTORY

Chronic Illness:_______________
Surgery:_______________
Allergy:_______________
Communicable Disease:_______________

FAMILY HISTORY

Type of Family:
Nuclear: _______________ Number of Persons: _______________
Joint: _______________ Number of Persons: _______________

DISEASES: Chronic Illness

Hypertension:________ Diabetes:________ Genetic Diseases:________ Psychiatric Disorders:________
Others : _______________

HISTORY OF MULTIPLE BIRTHS

Number of Children :__________ Girl Child:__________ Boy Child__________

SOCIOECONOMIC BACKGROUND

Religion:_______________ Family Income:_______________
Education: Husband: _______________ Wife: _______________
Occupation: Husband: _______________ Wife: _______________

MENSTRUAL HISTORY

Menarchy:__________ Duration:__________ Interval:__________ Flow:__________

MARITAL HISTORY

Age of Marriage:_______________
Consanguineous: Yes/No

DIETARY PATTERN

Vegetarian: _______________ Nonvegetarian: _______________
Likes:_______________ Dislikes:_______________
Habits: Smoking/Drinking Alchohol/Chewing Pan/Tobacco

PAST OBSTETRICAL HISTORY

S.No	Year	Full Term	Abortion	Type of Delivery	Sex of Baby	Alive	Stillbirth	Weight	Remarks

PRESENT PREGNANCY

Admission Notes:

Admission on:____________ at:____________ Contractions Commenced:____________ at:____________

Period of Gestation:____________ Membranes: Intact:____________ Ruptured on:____________

Height of Fundus: ____________ Contractions ____________

Presentation:____________ Position:____________

Engaged/Nonengaged: ____________ FHR: ____________

Bladder:____________ Bowel:____________

BP:____________ TPR: ____________

Special Observations: ____________

PRENATAL VISITS

Date of Booking	Weight	Height	Urine		BP	FHR	Weeks of Gestation	Height of Fundus	Position	Treatment
			Protein	Glucose						

EXAMINATION AND INVESTIGATIONS

Blood Group:________ Rh Factor:________ Hb:________ VDRL:________ HIV:________ Others:________

Heart________ Lungs________ Breast________ Abdomen________ Perineum________

DELIVERY RECORD

Onset of True Labour: Date:____________ Time:____________

Time of Full Dilatation: Date:____________ Time:____________

Membranes Ruptured at:____________ Spontaneous/Artificial: ____________ PROM:____________

THE SIMPLIFIED PARTOGRAPH

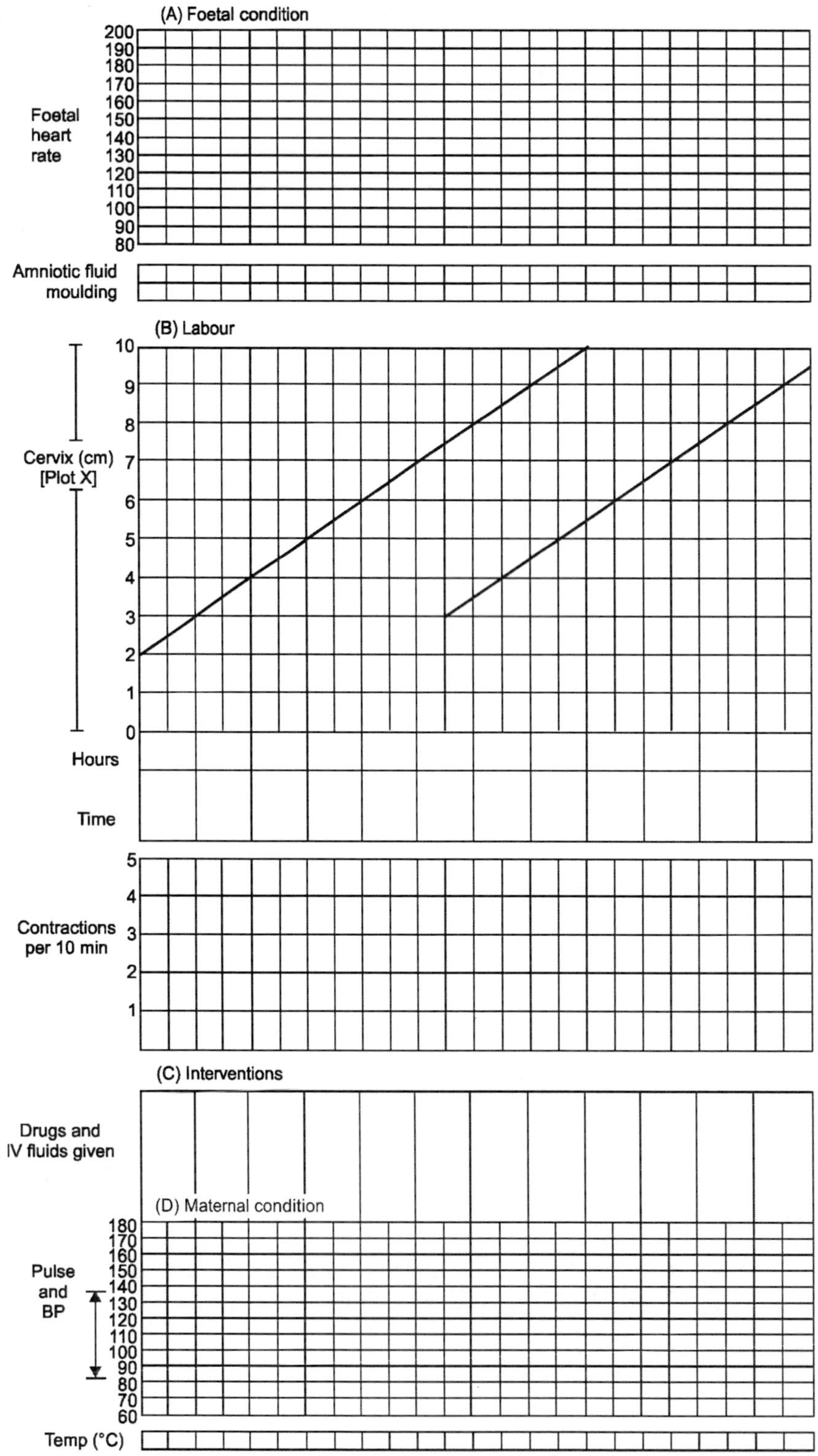

a. Delivery of Baby

Baby Born at:______________ AM/PM, Male/Female:______________________ Mode of Delivery: __________________
Condition of Baby: Active/ Nonactive/Asphyxiated ____

b. Delivery of Placenta and Membranes

Delivery at:___________________________________ AM/PM
Spontaneously/Manually Removed ____
Typeofplacenta____
PlacentaandMembranes: Complete/ Incomplete____
Weight_______________Cord Length_______________________Any Abnormality_________________________

c. Blood Loss (Approximate Total Amount)

Before Delivery of the Placenta__________________________ ml
During Delivery of the Placenta__________________________ml
After Delivery of the Placenta____________________________ml
Total Amount_________________________ ml

d. Perineum

Intact___________________Episiotomy____________________Laceration__________________Repair_______________

e. Medicationsgiven____

f. Length of Labour

Duration of Labour

Progress of Labour	Date	Time	Total...... Hrs..... Min.....
Contraction Started			...... Hrs..... Min.....
Full Dilatation			
Delivery of Baby			...... Hrs..... Min.....
Delivery of Placenta			...... Hrs..... Min.....
Total Time Taken for Labour			

Condition of the Mother following Delivery

Pulse_______________BP__________________ Height of Uterus_______________ Vaginal Bleeding______________________
Breastfeeding Initiated at ____

Sign of Supervisor **Sign of Student**

INTRANATAL CASE STUDY

Name:__________ Age: __________ G, P, L, A __________
Name of the Hospital:__________ Hospital Number: __________
Date of Admission:__________

ANTENATAL RECORD

Date of Booking:__________ LMP:__________ EDD:__________ Gestation at 1st Visit:__________

MEDICAL HISTORY

Chronic Illness:__________
Surgery:__________
Allergy:__________
Communicable Disease:__________

FAMILY HISTORY

Type of Family:
Nuclear: __________ Number of Persons: __________
Joint: __________ Number of Persons: __________

DISEASES: Chronic Illness

Hypertension:__________ Diabetes:__________ Genetic Diseases:__________ Psychiatric Disorders:__________
Others : __________

HISTORY OF MULTIPLE BIRTHS

Number of Children :__________ Girl Child:__________ Boy Child__________

SOCIOECONOMIC BACKGROUND

Religion:__________ Family Income:__________
Education: Husband: __________ Wife: __________
Occupation: Husband: __________ Wife: __________

MENSTRUAL HISTORY

Menarchy:__________ Duration:__________ Interval:__________ Flow:__________

MARITAL HISTORY

Age of Marriage:__________
Consanguineous: Yes/No

DIETARY PATTERN

Vegetarian: __________ Nonvegetarian: __________
Likes:__________ Dislikes:__________
Habits: Smoking/Drinking Alchohol/Chewing Pan/Tobacco

PAST OBSTETRICAL HISTORY

S.No	Year	Full Term	Abortion	Type of Delivery	Sex of Baby	Alive	Stillbirth	Weight	Remarks

PRESENT PREGNANCY

Admission Notes:

Admission on:__________ at: __________ Contractions Commenced:__________ at:__________

Period of Gestation:__________ Membranes: Intact:__________ Ruptured on:__________

Height of Fundus: __________ Contractions __________

Presentation:__________ Position:__________

Engaged/Nonengaged: __________ FHR: __________

Bladder :__________ Bowel:__________

BP:__________ TPR: __________

Special Observations: __________

PRENATAL VISITS

Date of Booking	Weight	Height	Urine		BP	FHR	Weeks of Gestation	Height of Fundus	Position	Treatment
			Protein	Glucose						

EXAMINATION AND INVESTIGATIONS

Blood Group:________ Rh Factor:________ Hb:________ VDRL:________ HIV:________ Others:________

Heart________ Lungs________ Breast________ Abdomen________ Perineum________

DELIVERY RECORD

Onset of True Labour: Date:__________ Time:__________

Time of Full Dilatation: Date:__________ Time:__________

Membranes Ruptured at:__________ Spontaneous/Artificial: __________ PROM:__________

THE SIMPLIFIED PARTOGRAPH

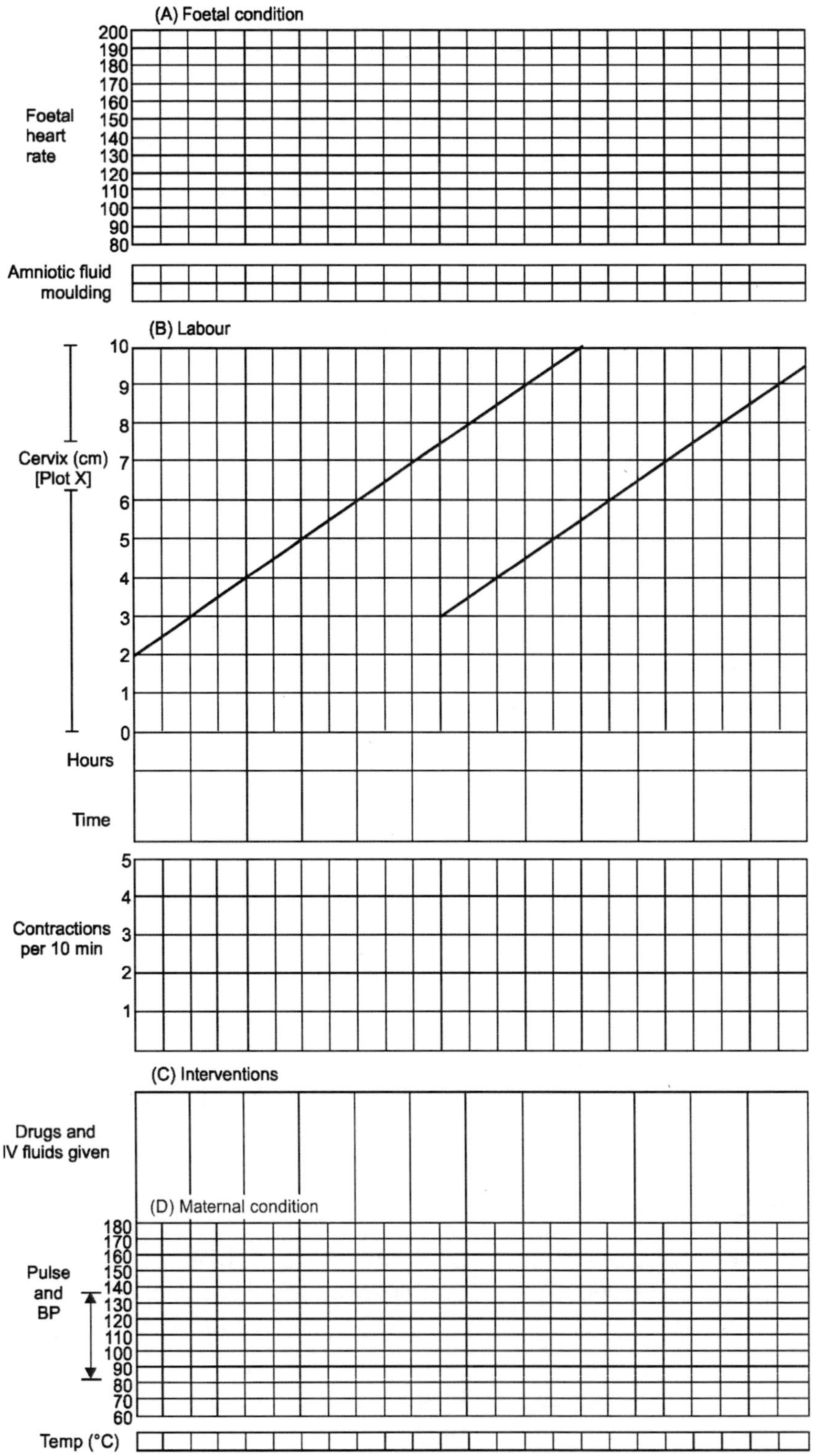

a. Delivery of Baby

Baby Born at:______________ AM/PM, Male/Female:____________________ Mode of Delivery: __________________
Condition of Baby: Active/ Nonactive/Asphyxiated ____

b. Delivery of Placenta and Membranes

Delivery at:__________________________________ AM/PM
Spontaneously/Manually Removed ____
Typeofplacenta____
PlacentaandMembranes: Complete/Incomplete____
Weight______________CordLength______________________AnyAbnormality______________________

c. Blood Loss (Approximate Total Amount)

Before Delivery of the Placenta_________________________ ml
During Delivery of the Placenta_________________________ml
After Delivery of the Placenta___________________________ml
Total Amount________________________ ml

d. Perineum

Intact__________________Episiotomy___________________Laceration__________________Repair_______________

e. Medicationsgiven____

f. Length of Labour

Duration of Labour

Progress of Labour	Date	Time	Total...... Hrs..... Min.....
Contraction Started			...... Hrs..... Min.....
Full Dilatation			
Delivery of Baby			...... Hrs..... Min.....
Delivery of Placenta			...... Hrs..... Min.....
Total Time Taken for Labour			

Condition of the Mother following Delivery

Pulse______________BP__________________ Height of Uterus______________ Vaginal Bleeding______________________
Breastfeeding Initiated at ____

Sign of Supervisor **Sign of Student**

INTRANATAL CASE STUDY

Name:____________________ Age: __________ G, P, L, A ____________________
Name of the Hospital:____________________ Hospital Number: ____________________
Date of Admission:____________________

ANTENATAL RECORD

Date of Booking:__________ LMP:__________ EDD:__________ Gestation at 1st Visit:__________

MEDICAL HISTORY

Chronic Illness:____________________
Surgery:____________________
Allergy:____________________
Communicable Disease:____________________

FAMILY HISTORY

Type of Family:
Nuclear: ____________________ Number of Persons: ____________________
Joint: ____________________ Number of Persons: ____________________

DISEASES: Chronic Illness

Hypertension:__________ Diabetes:__________ Genetic Diseases:__________ Psychiatric Disorders:__________
Others : ____________________

HISTORY OF MULTIPLE BIRTHS

Number of Children :__________ Girl Child:__________ Boy Child__________

SOCIOECONOMIC BACKGROUND

Religion:____________________ Family Income:____________________
Education: Husband: ____________________ Wife: ____________________
Occupation: Husband: ____________________ Wife: ____________________

MENSTRUAL HISTORY

Menarchy:__________ Duration:__________ Interval:__________ Flow:__________

MARITAL HISTORY

Age of Marriage:____________________
Consanguineous: Yes/No

DIETARY PATTERN

Vegetarian: ____________________ Nonvegetarian: ____________________
Likes:____________________ Dislikes:____________________
Habits: Smoking/Drinking Alchohol/Chewing Pan/Tobacco

PAST OBSTETRICAL HISTORY

S.No	Year	Full Term	Abortion	Type of Delivery	Sex of Baby	Alive	Stillbirth	Weight	Remarks

PRESENT PREGNANCY

Admission Notes:

Admission on:____________ at: ______________ Contractions Commenced:________________ at:__________________

Period of Gestation:______________________ Membranes: Intact:____________________ Ruptured on:________________

Height of Fundus: _________________________________ Contractions ______________________________________

Presentation:_______________________________________ Position:____

Engaged/Nonengaged: ____________________________________ FHR: ____

Bladder :____ Bowel:____________________________________

BP:____ TPR: _______________________________________

Special Observations: ____

PRENATAL VISITS

Date of Booking	Weight	Height	Urine		BP	FHR	Weeks of Gestation	Height of Fundus	Position	Treatment
			Protein	Glucose						

EXAMINATION AND INVESTIGATIONS

Blood Group:________ Rh Factor:__________ Hb:__________ VDRL:__________ HIV:__________Others:________________

Heart_________ Lungs____________ Breast______________ Abdomen________________ Perineum__________________

DELIVERY RECORD

Onset of True Labour: Date:________________________ Time:________________________

Time of Full Dilatation: Date:______________________ Time:________________________

Membranes Ruptured at:______________________ Spontaneous/Artificial: ______________ PROM:__________________

THE SIMPLIFIED PARTOGRAPH

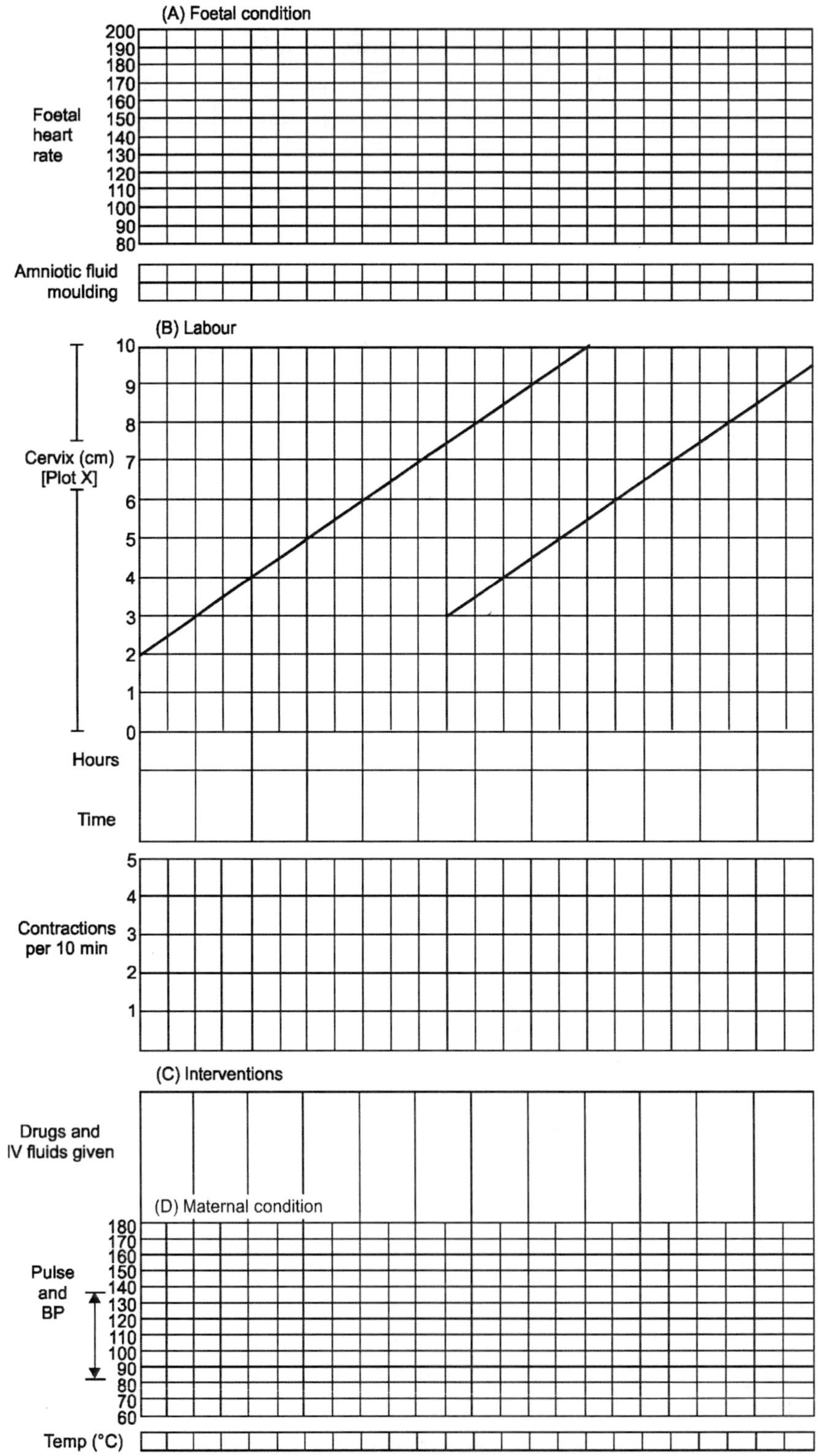

a. Delivery of Baby

Baby Born at:______________ AM/PM, Male/Female:______________________ Mode of Delivery: __________________
Condition of Baby: Active/ Nonactive/Asphyxiated ____

b. Delivery of Placenta and Membranes

Delivery at:___________________________________ AM/PM
Spontaneously/Manually Removed ____
Typeofplacenta____
PlacentaandMembranes: Complete/Incomplete____
Weight______________CordLength______________________AnyAbnormality_________________________

c. Blood Loss (Approximate Total Amount)

Before Delivery of the Placenta_________________________ ml
During Delivery of the Placenta_________________________ml
After Delivery of the Placenta__________________________ml
Total Amount________________________ ml

d. Perineum

Intact__________________Episiotomy___________________Laceration__________________Repair_______________

e. Medicationsgiven____

f. Length of Labour

Duration of Labour

Progress of Labour	Date	Time	Total...... Hrs..... Min.....
Contraction Started			...... Hrs..... Min.....
Full Dilatation			
Delivery of Baby			...... Hrs..... Min.....
Delivery of Placenta			...... Hrs..... Min.....
Total Time Taken for Labour			

Condition of the Mother following Delivery

Pulse______________BP_________________ Height of Uterus______________ Vaginal Bleeding_____________________
Breastfeeding Initiated at ____

Sign of Supervisor **Sign of Student**

INTRANATAL CASE STUDY

Name:______________________ Age: __________ G, P, L, A ______________________
Name of the Hospital:______________________ Hospital Number: ______________________
Date of Admission:______________________

ANTENATAL RECORD

Date of Booking:______________ LMP:__________ EDD:__________ Gestation at 1st Visit:______________

MEDICAL HISTORY

Chronic Illness:______________________
Surgery:______________________
Allergy:______________________
Communicable Disease:______________________

FAMILY HISTORY

Type of Family:
Nuclear: ______________________ Number of Persons: ______________________
Joint: ______________________ Number of Persons: ______________________

DISEASES: Chronic Illness

Hypertension:__________ Diabetes:__________ Genetic Diseases:__________ Psychiatric Disorders:__________
Others : ______________________

HISTORY OF MULTIPLE BIRTHS

Number of Children :______________ Girl Child:______________ Boy Child______________

SOCIOECONOMIC BACKGROUND

Religion:______________________ Family Income:______________________
Education: Husband: ______________________ Wife: ______________________
Occupation: Husband: ______________________ Wife: ______________________

MENSTRUAL HISTORY

Menarchy:______________ Duration:______________ Interval:______________ Flow:______________

MARITAL HISTORY

Age of Marriage:______________
Consanguineous: Yes/No

DIETARY PATTERN

Vegetarian: ______________________ Nonvegetarian: ______________________
Likes:______________________ Dislikes:______________________
Habits: Smoking/Drinking Alchohol/Chewing Pan/Tobacco

PAST OBSTETRICAL HISTORY

S.No	Year	Full Term	Abortion	Type of Delivery	Sex of Baby	Alive	Stillbirth	Weight	Remarks

PRESENT PREGNANCY

Admission Notes:

Admission on:____________ at:____________ Contractions Commenced:______________ at:____________________

Period of Gestation:____________________ Membranes: Intact:____________________ Ruptured on:________________

Height of Fundus: ______________________________ Contractions ____

Presentation:____________________________________ Position:____

Engaged/Nonengaged: ___________________________________ FHR: ____________________________________

Bladder :____ Bowel:________________________________

BP:____ TPR: __________________________________

Special Observations: ____

PRENATAL VISITS

Date of Booking	Weight	Height	Urine		BP	FHR	Weeks of Gestation	Height of Fundus	Position	Treatment
			Protein	Glucose						

EXAMINATION AND INVESTIGATIONS

Blood Group:________ Rh Factor:_________ Hb:__________ VDRL:__________ HIV:__________Others:______________

Heart_________ Lungs____________ Breast_____________ Abdomen_______________ Perineum_________________

DELIVERY RECORD

Onset of True Labour: Date:______________________ Time:______________________

Time of Full Dilatation: Date:_____________________ Time:______________________

Membranes Ruptured at:_____________________ Spontaneous/Artificial: _____________ PROM:________________

THE SIMPLIFIED PARTOGRAPH

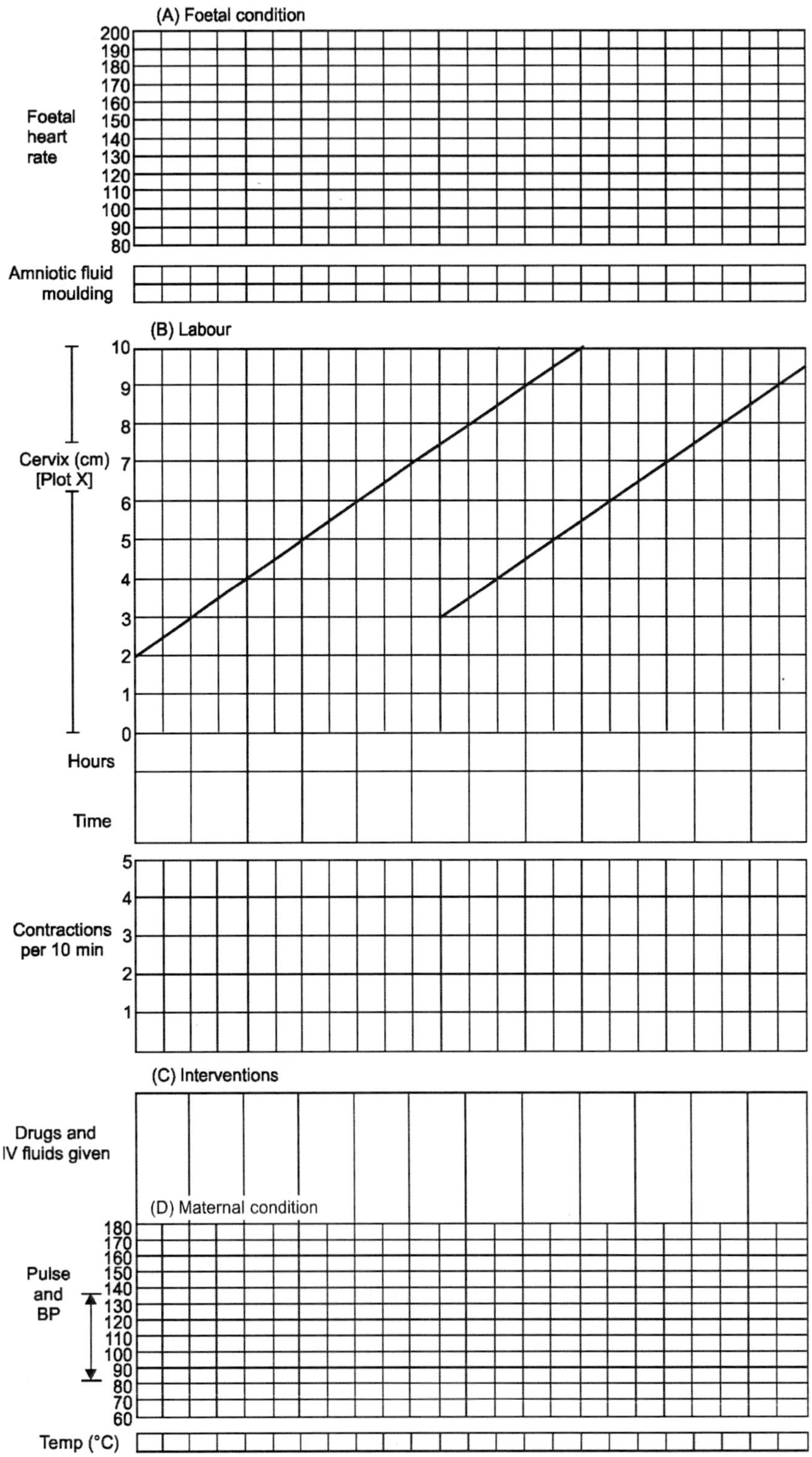

a. Delivery of Baby

Baby Born at:______________ AM/PM, Male/Female:______________________ Mode of Delivery: ___________________
Condition of Baby: Active/ Nonactive/Asphyxiated ____

b. Delivery of Placenta and Membranes

Delivery at:___________________________________ AM/PM
Spontaneously/Manually Removed ____
Typeofplacenta____
PlacentaandMembranes: Complete/Incomplete____
Weight_______________Cord Length_______________________Any Abnormality_________________________

c. Blood Loss (Approximate Total Amount)

Before Delivery of the Placenta__________________________ ml
During Delivery of the Placenta__________________________ml
After Delivery of the Placenta____________________________ml
Total Amount_________________________ ml

d. Perineum

Intact___________________Episiotomy____________________Laceration___________________Repair________________

e. Medicationsgiven____

f. Length of Labour

Duration of Labour

Progress of Labour	Date	Time	Total...... Hrs..... Min.....
Contraction Started			...... Hrs..... Min.....
Full Dilatation			
Delivery of Baby			...... Hrs..... Min.....
Delivery of Placenta			...... Hrs..... Min.....
Total Time Taken for Labour			

Condition of the Mother following Delivery

Pulse_______________BP__________________ Height of Uterus_______________ Vaginal Bleeding______________________
Breastfeeding Initiated at ____

Sign of Supervisor **Sign of Student**

INTRANATAL CASE STUDY

Name:__________ Age: __________ G, P, L, A __________
Name of the Hospital:__________ Hospital Number: __________
Date of Admission:__________

ANTENATAL RECORD

Date of Booking:__________ LMP:__________ EDD:__________ Gestation at 1st Visit:__________

MEDICAL HISTORY

Chronic Illness:__________
Surgery:__________
Allergy:__________
Communicable Disease:__________

FAMILY HISTORY

Type of Family:
Nuclear: __________ Number of Persons: __________
Joint: __________ Number of Persons: __________

DISEASES: Chronic Illness

Hypertension:__________ Diabetes:__________ Genetic Diseases:__________ Psychiatric Disorders:__________
Others : __________

HISTORY OF MULTIPLE BIRTHS

Number of Children :__________ Girl Child:__________ Boy Child__________

SOCIOECONOMIC BACKGROUND

Religion:__________ Family Income:__________
Education: Husband: __________ Wife: __________
Occupation: Husband: __________ Wife: __________

MENSTRUAL HISTORY

Menarchy:__________ Duration:__________ Interval:__________ Flow:__________

MARITAL HISTORY

Age of Marriage:__________
Consanguineous: Yes/No

DIETARY PATTERN

Vegetarian: __________ Nonvegetarian: __________
Likes:__________ Dislikes:__________
Habits: Smoking/Drinking Alchohol/Chewing Pan/Tobacco

PAST OBSTETRICAL HISTORY

S.No	Year	Full Term	Abortion	Type of Delivery	Sex of Baby	Alive	Stillbirth	Weight	Remarks

PRESENT PREGNANCY

Admission Notes:

Admission on:____________ at:_____________ Contractions Commenced:________________ at:____________________

Period of Gestation:______________________ Membranes: Intact:_____________________ Ruptured on:______________

Height of Fundus: _______________________________ Contractions ______________________________________

Presentation:____ Position:_____________________________________

Engaged/Nonengaged: _____________________________________ FHR: _______________________________________

Bladder :____ Bowel:____________________________________

BP:____ TPR: ____

Special Observations: ____

PRENATAL VISITS

Date of Booking	Weight	Height	Urine		BP	FHR	Weeks of Gestation	Height of Fundus	Position	Treatment
			Protein	Glucose						

EXAMINATION AND INVESTIGATIONS

Blood Group:________ Rh Factor:_________ Hb:__________ VDRL:__________ HIV:__________Others:______________

Heart_________ Lungs_____________ Breast______________ Abdomen________________ Perineum__________________

DELIVERY RECORD

Onset of True Labour: Date:________________________ Time:_______________________

Time of Full Dilatation: Date:______________________ Time:_______________________

Membranes Ruptured at:_____________________ Spontaneous/Artificial: ______________ PROM:__________________

THE SIMPLIFIED PARTOGRAPH

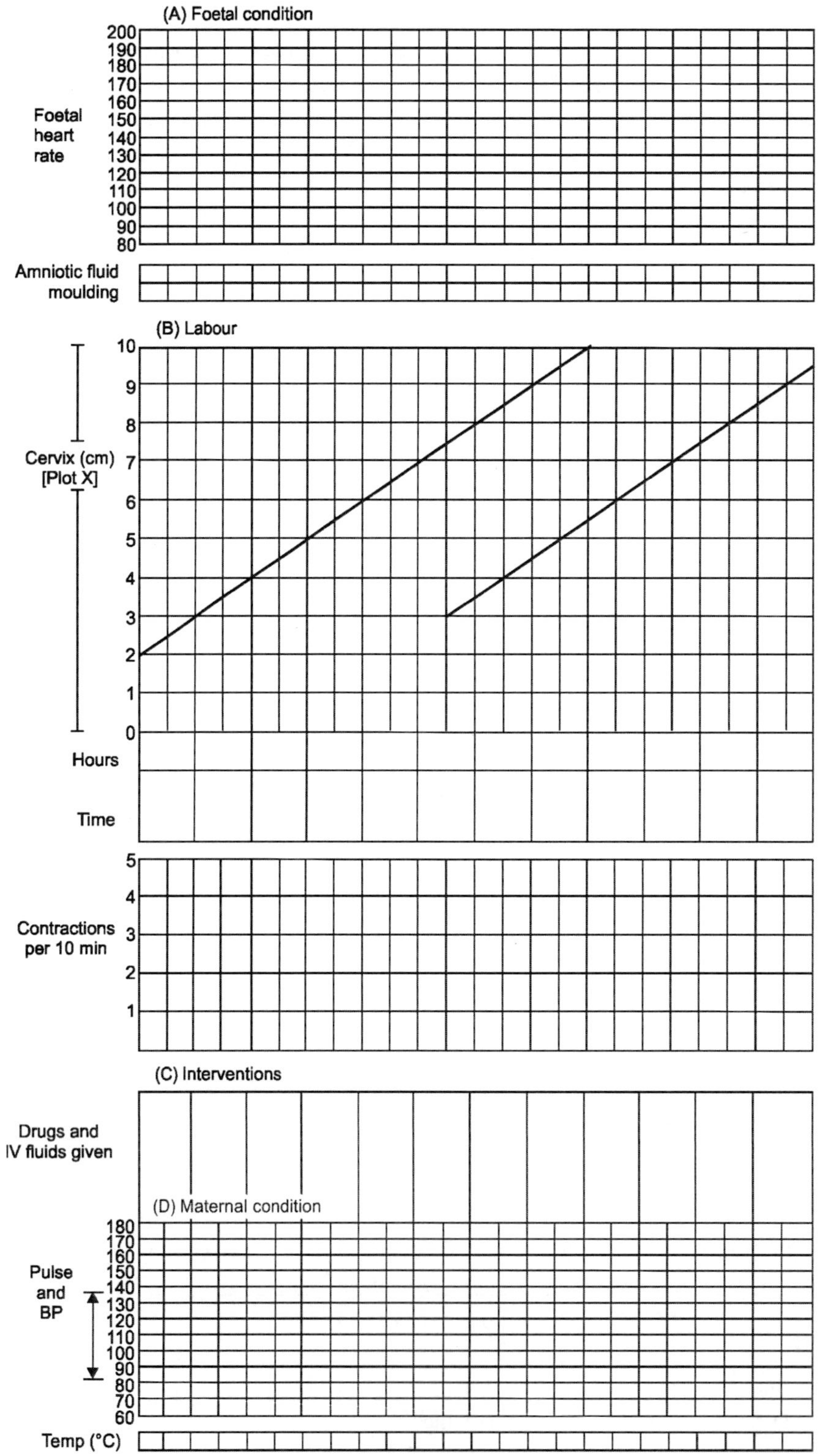

a. Delivery of Baby

Baby Born at:______________ AM/PM, Male/Female:______________________ Mode of Delivery: __________________
Condition of Baby: Active/ Nonactive/Asphyxiated ____

b. Delivery of Placenta and Membranes

Delivery at:___________________________________ AM/PM
Spontaneously/Manually Removed ____
Typeofplacenta____
PlacentaandMembranes: Complete/Incomplete____
Weight______________CordLength_______________________AnyAbnormality_______________________

c. Blood Loss (Approximate Total Amount)

Before Delivery of the Placenta__________________________ ml
During Delivery of the Placenta__________________________ml
After Delivery of the Placenta____________________________ml
Total Amount_________________________ ml

d. Perineum

Intact__________________Episiotomy___________________Laceration__________________Repair_______________

e. Medicationsgiven____

f. Length of Labour

Duration of Labour

Progress of Labour	Date	Time	Total...... Hrs..... Min.....
Contraction Started			...... Hrs..... Min.....
Full Dilatation			
Delivery of Baby			...... Hrs..... Min.....
Delivery of Placenta			...... Hrs..... Min.....
Total Time Taken for Labour			

Condition of the Mother following Delivery

Pulse______________BP_________________ Height of Uterus______________ Vaginal Bleeding______________________
Breastfeeding Initiated at ____

Sign of Supervisor **Sign of Student**

INTRANATAL CASE STUDY

Name:____________________________ Age: __________ G, P, L, A ________________________
Name of the Hospital:________________________ Hospital Number: ________________________
Date of Admission:________________________

ANTENATAL RECORD

Date of Booking:_____________ LMP:_________ EDD:__________ Gestation at 1st Visit:__________

MEDICAL HISTORY

Chronic Illness:____
Surgery:____
Allergy:____
Communicable Disease:____

FAMILY HISTORY

Type of Family:
Nuclear: ________________________ Number of Persons: ____________________
Joint: __________________________ Number of Persons: ____________________

DISEASES: Chronic Illness

Hypertension:_________ Diabetes:_______ Genetic Diseases:________ Psychiatric Disorders:________
Others : ____

HISTORY OF MULTIPLE BIRTHS

Number of Children :______________ Girl Child:_______________ Boy Child________________

SOCIOECONOMIC BACKGROUND

Religion:_________________________ Family Income:______________________________
Education: Husband: _________________________ Wife: __________________________
Occupation: Husband: ____________________ Wife: __________________________________

MENSTRUAL HISTORY

Menarchy:_______________ Duration:__________ Interval:____________ Flow:___________

MARITAL HISTORY

Age of Marriage:__________________
Consanguineous: Yes/No

DIETARY PATTERN

Vegetarian: ________________________ Nonvegetarian: ______________________________
Likes:______________________________ Dislikes:__________________________________
Habits: Smoking/Drinking Alchohol/Chewing Pan/Tobacco

PAST OBSTETRICAL HISTORY

S.No	Year	Full Term	Abortion	Type of Delivery	Sex of Baby	Alive	Stillbirth	Weight	Remarks

PRESENT PREGNANCY

Admission Notes:

Admission on:____________ at:____________ Contractions Commenced:______________ at:__________________

Period of Gestation:____________________ Membranes: Intact:_________________ Ruptured on:_______________

Height of Fundus: ______________________________ Contractions ______________________________________

–

Presentation:____________________________________ Position:____

Engaged/Nonengaged: _________________________________ FHR: ____

Bladder:____ Bowel:____

BP:____ TPR: ____

Special Observations: ____

PRENATAL VISITS

Date of Booking	Weight	Height	Urine		BP	FHR	Weeks of Gestation	Height of Fundus	Position	Treatment
			Protein	Glucose						

EXAMINATION AND INVESTIGATIONS

Blood Group:________ Rh Factor:_________ Hb:__________ VDRL:__________ HIV:__________ Others:______________

Heart_________ Lungs____________ Breast_____________ Abdomen________________ Perineum__________________

DELIVERY RECORD

Onset of True Labour: Date:_______________________ Time:______________________

Time of Full Dilatation: Date:_______________________ Time:______________________

Membranes Ruptured at:_____________________ Spontaneous/Artificial: ______________ PROM:__________________

THE SIMPLIFIED PARTOGRAPH

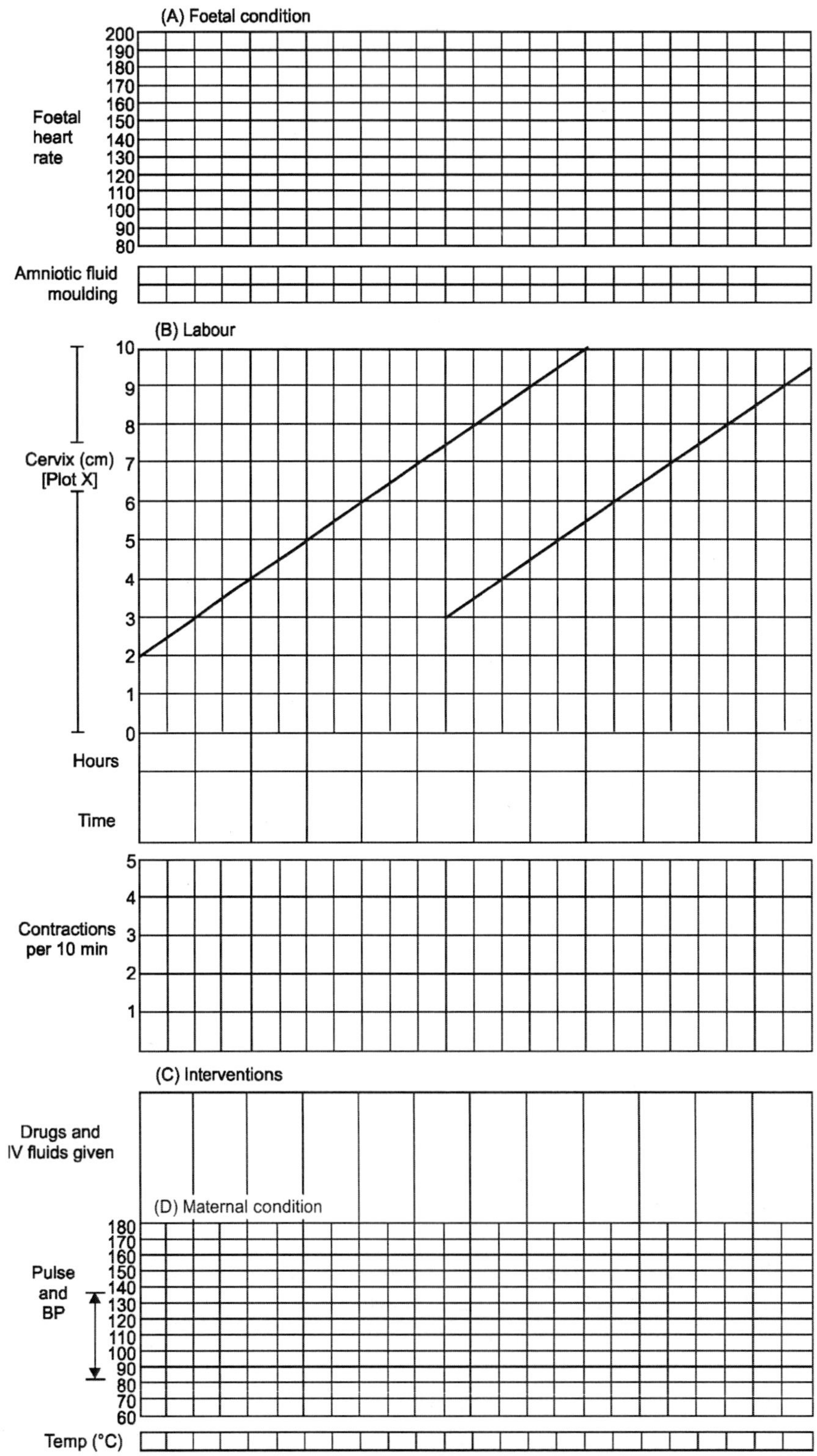

a. Delivery of Baby

Baby Born at:__________ AM/PM, Male/Female:__________ Mode of Delivery: __________
Condition of Baby: Active/ Nonactive/Asphyxiated __________

b. Delivery of Placenta and Membranes

Delivery at:__________ AM/PM
Spontaneously/Manually Removed __________
Typeofplacenta__________
PlacentaandMembranes: Complete/Incomplete__________
Weight__________CordLength__________AnyAbnormality__________

c. Blood Loss (Approximate Total Amount)

Before Delivery of the Placenta__________ ml
During Delivery of the Placenta__________ml
After Delivery of the Placenta__________ml
Total Amount__________ ml

d. Perineum

Intact__________Episiotomy__________Laceration__________Repair__________

e. Medicationsgiven__________

f. Length of Labour

Duration of Labour

Progress of Labour	Date	Time	Total...... Hrs..... Min.....
Contraction Started			...... Hrs..... Min.....
Full Dilatation			
Delivery of Baby			...... Hrs..... Min.....
Delivery of Placenta			...... Hrs..... Min.....
Total Time Taken for Labour			

Condition of the Mother following Delivery

Pulse__________BP__________ Height of Uterus__________ Vaginal Bleeding__________
Breastfeeding Initiated at __________

Sign of Supervisor **Sign of Student**

INTRANATAL CASE STUDY

Name:____________________ Age: __________ G, P, L, A ____________________
Name of the Hospital:____________________ Hospital Number: ____________________
Date of Admission:____________________

ANTENATAL RECORD

Date of Booking:__________ LMP:__________ EDD:__________ Gestation at 1st Visit:__________

MEDICAL HISTORY

Chronic Illness:____________________
Surgery:____________________
Allergy:____________________
Communicable Disease:____________________

FAMILY HISTORY

Type of Family:
Nuclear: ____________________ Number of Persons: ____________________
Joint: ____________________ Number of Persons: ____________________

DISEASES: Chronic Illness

Hypertension:__________ Diabetes:__________ Genetic Diseases:__________ Psychiatric Disorders:__________
Others : ____________________

HISTORY OF MULTIPLE BIRTHS

Number of Children :__________ Girl Child:__________ Boy Child__________

SOCIOECONOMIC BACKGROUND

Religion:____________________ Family Income:____________________
Education: Husband: ____________________ Wife: ____________________
Occupation: Husband: ____________________ Wife: ____________________

MENSTRUAL HISTORY

Menarchy:__________ Duration:__________ Interval:__________ Flow:__________

MARITAL HISTORY

Age of Marriage:____________________
Consanguineous: Yes/No

DIETARY PATTERN

Vegetarian: ____________________ Nonvegetarian: ____________________
Likes:____________________ Dislikes:____________________
Habits: Smoking/Drinking Alchohol/Chewing Pan/Tobacco

PAST OBSTETRICAL HISTORY

S.No	Year	Full Term	Abortion	Type of Delivery	Sex of Baby	Alive	Stillbirth	Weight	Remarks

PRESENT PREGNANCY

Admission Notes:

Admission on:__________ at:__________ Contractions Commenced:__________ at:__________
Period of Gestation:__________ Membranes: Intact:__________ Ruptured on:__________
Height of Fundus: __________ Contractions __________
Presentation:__________ Position:__________
Engaged/Nonengaged: __________ FHR: __________
Bladder :__________ Bowel:__________
BP:__________ TPR: __________
Special Observations: __________

PRENATAL VISITS

Date of Booking	Weight	Height	Urine		BP	FHR	Weeks of Gestation	Height of Fundus	Position	Treatment
			Protein	Glucose						

EXAMINATION AND INVESTIGATIONS

Blood Group:________ Rh Factor:________ Hb:________ VDRL:________ HIV:________ Others:________
Heart________ Lungs________ Breast________ Abdomen________ Perineum________

DELIVERY RECORD

Onset of True Labour: Date:__________ Time:__________
Time of Full Dilatation: Date:__________ Time:__________
Membranes Ruptured at:__________ Spontaneous/Artificial: __________ PROM:__________

THE SIMPLIFIED PARTOGRAPH

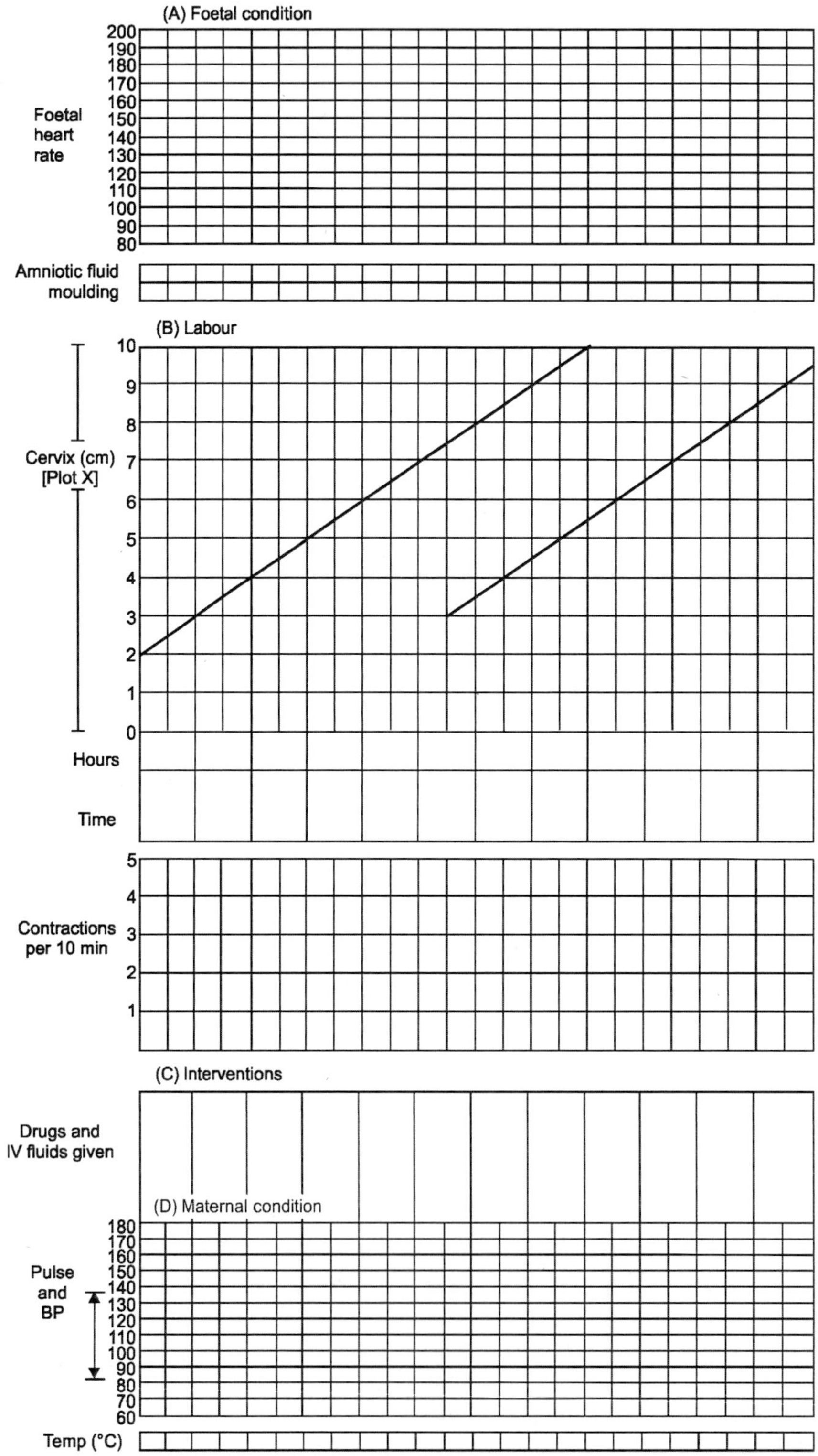

a. Delivery of Baby

Baby Born at:______________ AM/PM, Male/Female:_____________________ Mode of Delivery: __________________
Condition of Baby: Active/ Nonactive/Asphyxiated ____

b. Delivery of Placenta and Membranes

Delivery at:__________________________________ AM/PM
Spontaneously/Manually Removed ____
Typeofplacenta____
PlacentaandMembranes: Complete/Incomplete____
Weight______________CordLength______________________AnyAbnormality___________________

c. Blood Loss (Approximate Total Amount)

Before Delivery of the Placenta_________________________ ml
During Delivery of the Placenta_________________________ml
After Delivery of the Placenta___________________________ml
Total Amount________________________ ml

d. Perineum

Intact__________________Episiotomy___________________Laceration__________________Repair_______________

e. Medicationsgiven____

f. Length of Labour

Duration of Labour

Progress of Labour	Date	Time	Total...... Hrs..... Min.....
Contraction Started			...... Hrs..... Min.....
Full Dilatation			
Delivery of Baby			...... Hrs..... Min.....
Delivery of Placenta			...... Hrs..... Min.....
Total Time Taken for Labour			

Condition of the Mother following Delivery

Pulse______________BP_________________ Height of Uterus______________ Vaginal Bleeding______________________
Breastfeeding Initiated at ____

Sign of Supervisor **Sign of Student**

INTRANATAL CASE STUDY

Name:________________ Age: ________ G, P, L, A ________________
Name of the Hospital:________________ Hospital Number: ________________
Date of Admission:________________

ANTENATAL RECORD

Date of Booking:________ LMP:________ EDD:________ Gestation at 1st Visit:________

MEDICAL HISTORY

Chronic Illness:________________
Surgery:________________
Allergy:________________
Communicable Disease:________________

FAMILY HISTORY

Type of Family:
Nuclear: ________________ Number of Persons: ________________
Joint: ________________ Number of Persons: ________________

DISEASES: Chronic Illness

Hypertension:________ Diabetes:________ Genetic Diseases:________ Psychiatric Disorders:________
Others : ________________

HISTORY OF MULTIPLE BIRTHS

Number of Children :________ Girl Child:________ Boy Child________

SOCIOECONOMIC BACKGROUND

Religion:________________ Family Income:________________
Education: Husband: ________________ Wife: ________________
Occupation: Husband: ________________ Wife: ________________

MENSTRUAL HISTORY

Menarchy:________ Duration:________ Interval:________ Flow:________

MARITAL HISTORY

Age of Marriage:________________
Consanguineous: Yes/No

DIETARY PATTERN

Vegetarian: ________________ Nonvegetarian: ________________
Likes:________________ Dislikes:________________
Habits: Smoking/Drinking Alchohol/Chewing Pan/Tobacco

PAST OBSTETRICAL HISTORY

S.No	Year	Full Term	Abortion	Type of Delivery	Sex of Baby	Alive	Stillbirth	Weight	Remarks

PRESENT PREGNANCY

Admission Notes:

Admission on:____________ at: _____________ Contractions Commenced:________________ at:______________________

Period of Gestation:_____________________ Membranes: Intact:____________________ Ruptured on:________________

Height of Fundus: _______________________________ Contractions ____

Presentation:_____________________________________ Position:____

Engaged/Nonengaged: ____________________________________ FHR: _________________________________

Bladder :____ Bowel:______________________________

BP:____ TPR: _________________________________

Special Observations: ____

PRENATAL VISITS

Date of Booking	Weight	Height	Urine		BP	FHR	Weeks of Gestation	Height of Fundus	Position	Treatment
			Protein	Glucose						

EXAMINATION AND INVESTIGATIONS

Blood Group:________ Rh Factor:_________ Hb:__________ VDRL:__________ HIV:__________Others:________________

Heart_________ Lungs_____________ Breast_____________ Abdomen________________ Perineum__________________

DELIVERY RECORD

Onset of True Labour: Date:_______________________ Time:_______________________

Time of Full Dilatation: Date:_____________________ Time:_______________________

Membranes Ruptured at:______________________ Spontaneous/Artificial: ______________ PROM:___________________

THE SIMPLIFIED PARTOGRAPH

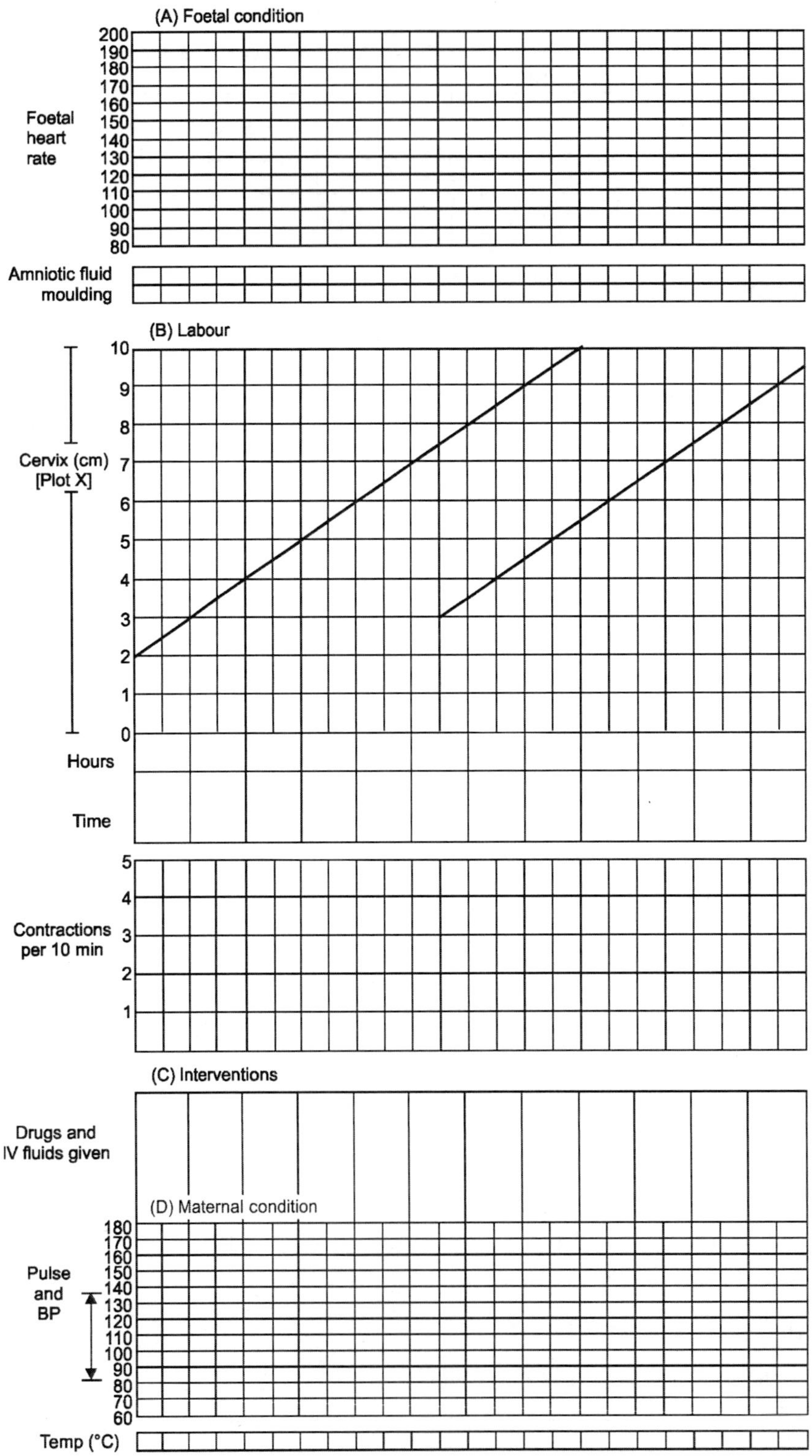

a. Delivery of Baby

Baby Born at:_____________ AM/PM, Male/Female:____________________ Mode of Delivery: _________________
Condition of Baby: Active/ Nonactive/Asphyxiated ____

b. Delivery of Placenta and Membranes

Delivery at:____________________________________ AM/PM
Spontaneously/Manually Removed ____
Typeofplacenta____
PlacentaandMembranes: Complete/ Incomplete____
Weight______________Cord Length______________________Any Abnormality________________________________

c. Blood Loss (Approximate Total Amount)

Before Delivery of the Placenta__________________________ ml
During Delivery of the Placenta__________________________ml
After Delivery of the Placenta____________________________ml
Total Amount_________________________ ml

d. Perineum

Intact__________________Episiotomy___________________Laceration__________________Repair_______________

e. Medicationsgiven____

f. Length of Labour

Duration of Labour

Progress of Labour	Date	Time	Total...... Hrs..... Min.....
Contraction Started			...... Hrs..... Min.....
Full Dilatation			
Delivery of Baby			...... Hrs..... Min.....
Delivery of Placenta			...... Hrs..... Min.....
Total Time Taken for Labour			

Condition of the Mother following Delivery

Pulse_______________BP_________________ Height of Uterus______________ Vaginal Bleeding______________________
Breastfeeding Initiated at ____

Sign of Supervisor **Sign of Student**

INTRANATAL CASE STUDY

Name:__________ Age: __________ G, P, L, A __________
Name of the Hospital:__________ Hospital Number: __________
Date of Admission:__________

ANTENATAL RECORD

Date of Booking:__________ LMP:__________ EDD:__________ Gestation at 1st Visit:__________

MEDICAL HISTORY

Chronic Illness:__________
Surgery:__________
Allergy:__________
Communicable Disease:__________

FAMILY HISTORY

Type of Family:
Nuclear: __________ Number of Persons: __________
Joint: __________ Number of Persons: __________

DISEASES: Chronic Illness

Hypertension:__________ Diabetes:__________ Genetic Diseases:__________ Psychiatric Disorders:__________
Others : __________

HISTORY OF MULTIPLE BIRTHS

Number of Children :__________ Girl Child:__________ Boy Child__________

SOCIOECONOMIC BACKGROUND

Religion:__________ Family Income:__________
Education: Husband: __________ Wife: __________
Occupation: Husband: __________ Wife: __________

MENSTRUAL HISTORY

Menarchy:__________ Duration:__________ Interval:__________ Flow:__________

MARITAL HISTORY

Age of Marriage:__________
Consanguineous: Yes/No

DIETARY PATTERN

Vegetarian: __________ Nonvegetarian: __________
Likes:__________ Dislikes:__________
Habits: Smoking/Drinking Alchohol/Chewing Pan/Tobacco

PAST OBSTETRICAL HISTORY

S.No	Year	Full Term	Abortion	Type of Delivery	Sex of Baby	Alive	Stillbirth	Weight	Remarks

PRESENT PREGNANCY

Admission Notes:

Admission on:_____________ at: ______________ Contractions Commenced:________________ at:______________________

Period of Gestation:______________________ Membranes: Intact:____________________ Ruptured on:________________

Height of Fundus: _________________________________ Contractions ___________________________________

Presentation:____________________________________ Position:___________________________________

Engaged/Nonengaged: _____________________________________ FHR: ____________________________

Bladder :____ Bowel:_____________________________

BP:____ TPR: _________________________________

Special Observations: ____

PRENATAL VISITS

Date of Booking	Weight	Height	Urine		BP	FHR	Weeks of Gestation	Height of Fundus	Position	Treatment
			Protein	Glucose						

EXAMINATION AND INVESTIGATIONS

Blood Group:________ Rh Factor:_________ Hb:___________ VDRL:__________ HIV:__________Others:_______________

Heart_________ Lungs_____________ Breast______________ Abdomen________________ Perineum__________________

DELIVERY RECORD

Onset of True Labour: Date:_______________________ Time:_______________________

Time of Full Dilatation: Date:_____________________ Time:_______________________

Membranes Ruptured at:______________________ Spontaneous/Artificial: ______________ PROM:__________________

THE SIMPLIFIED PARTOGRAPH

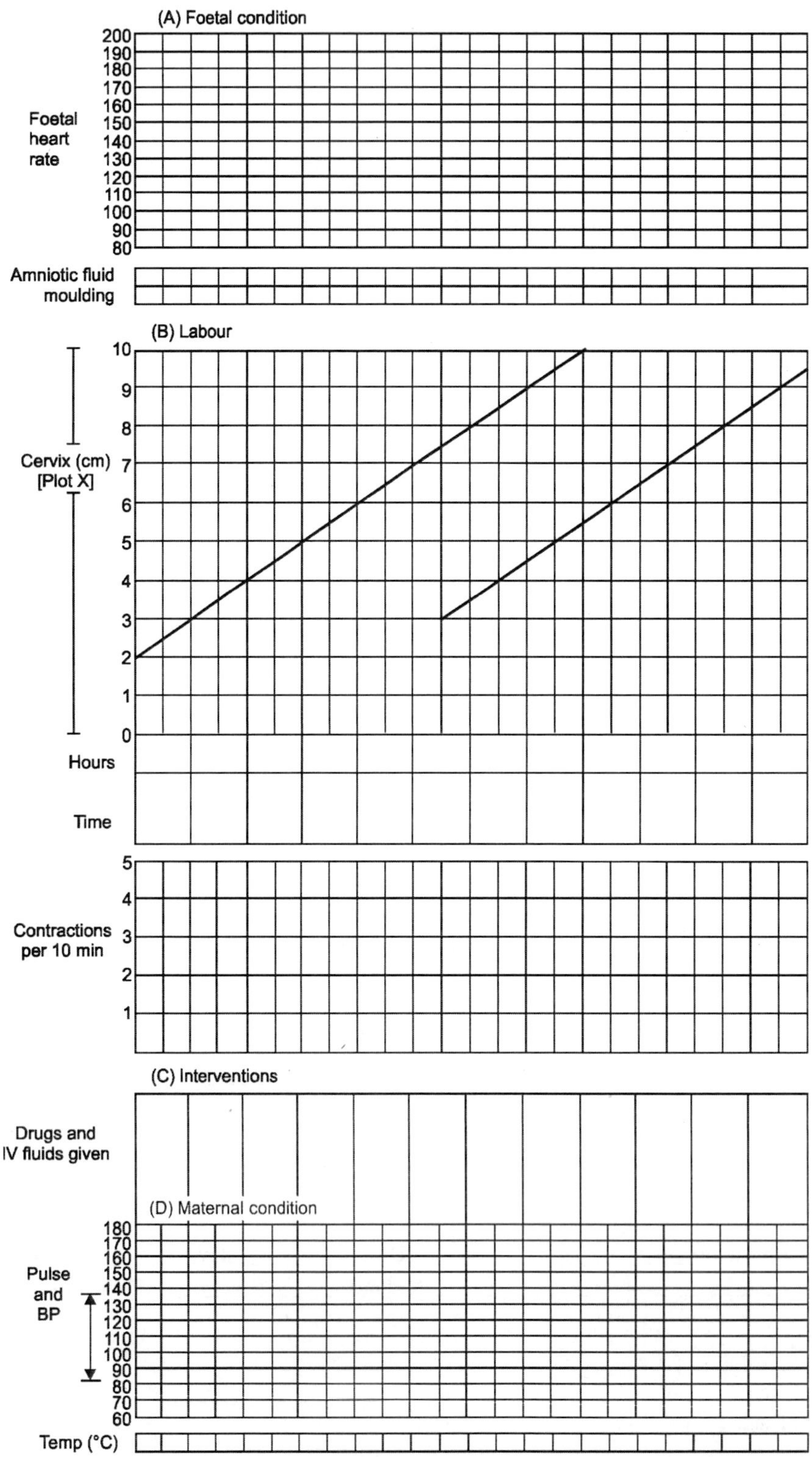

a. Delivery of Baby

Baby Born at:______________ AM/PM, Male/Female:_____________________ Mode of Delivery: __________________
Condition of Baby: Active/ Nonactive/Asphyxiated ____

b. Delivery of Placenta and Membranes

Delivery at:___________________________________ AM/PM
Spontaneously/Manually Removed ____
Typeofplacenta____
PlacentaandMembranes: Complete/Incomplete____
Weight______________Cord Length______________________Any Abnormality_____________________________

c. Blood Loss (Approximate Total Amount)

Before Delivery of the Placenta_________________________ ml
During Delivery of the Placenta_________________________ml
After Delivery of the Placenta___________________________ml
Total Amount________________________ ml

d. Perineum

Intact__________________Episiotomy___________________Laceration__________________Repair_______________

e. Medicationsgiven____

f. Length of Labour

Duration of Labour

Progress of Labour	Date	Time	Total...... Hrs..... Min.....
Contraction Started			...... Hrs..... Min.....
Full Dilatation			
Delivery of Baby			...... Hrs..... Min.....
Delivery of Placenta			...... Hrs..... Min.....
Total Time Taken for Labour			

Condition of the Mother following Delivery

Pulse______________BP_________________ Height of Uterus______________ Vaginal Bleeding______________________
Breastfeeding Initiated at ____

Sign of Supervisor **Sign of Student**

INTRANATAL CASE STUDY

Name:__________ Age: __________ G, P, L, A __________
Name of the Hospital:__________ Hospital Number: __________
Date of Admission:__________

ANTENATAL RECORD

Date of Booking:__________ LMP:__________ EDD:__________ Gestation at 1st Visit:__________

MEDICAL HISTORY

Chronic Illness:__________
Surgery:__________
Allergy:__________
Communicable Disease:__________

FAMILY HISTORY

Type of Family:
Nuclear: __________ Number of Persons: __________
Joint: __________ Number of Persons: __________

DISEASES: Chronic Illness

Hypertension:__________ Diabetes:__________ Genetic Diseases:__________ Psychiatric Disorders:__________
Others : __________

HISTORY OF MULTIPLE BIRTHS

Number of Children :__________ Girl Child:__________ Boy Child__________

SOCIOECONOMIC BACKGROUND

Religion:__________ Family Income:__________
Education: Husband: __________ Wife: __________
Occupation: Husband: __________ Wife: __________

MENSTRUAL HISTORY

Menarchy:__________ Duration:__________ Interval:__________ Flow:__________

MARITAL HISTORY

Age of Marriage:__________
Consanguineous: Yes/No

DIETARY PATTERN

Vegetarian: __________ Nonvegetarian: __________
Likes:__________ Dislikes:__________
Habits: Smoking/Drinking Alchohol/Chewing Pan/Tobacco

PAST OBSTETRICAL HISTORY

S.No	Year	Full Term	Abortion	Type of Delivery	Sex of Baby	Alive	Stillbirth	Weight	Remarks

PRESENT PREGNANCY

Admission Notes:

Admission on:_____________ at: ______________ Contractions Commenced:________________ at:______________________
Period of Gestation:______________________ Membranes: Intact:_____________________ Ruptured on:________________
Height of Fundus: _________________________________ Contractions ____
Presentation:____ Position:____
Engaged/Nonengaged: ______________________________________ FHR: ______________________________________
Bladder :____ Bowel:_____________________________
BP:____ TPR: ____________________________________
Special Observations: ____

PRENATAL VISITS

Date of Booking	Weight	Height	Urine		BP	FHR	Weeks of Gestation	Height of Fundus	Position	Treatment
			Protein	Glucose						

EXAMINATION AND INVESTIGATIONS

Blood Group:________ Rh Factor:_________ Hb:__________ VDRL:__________ HIV:__________Others:________________
Heart_________ Lungs_____________ Breast______________ Abdomen________________ Perineum__________________

DELIVERY RECORD

Onset of True Labour: Date:__________________________ Time:___________________________
Time of Full Dilatation: Date:________________________ Time:___________________________
Membranes Ruptured at:_________________________ Spontaneous/Artificial: _______________ PROM:___________________

THE SIMPLIFIED PARTOGRAPH

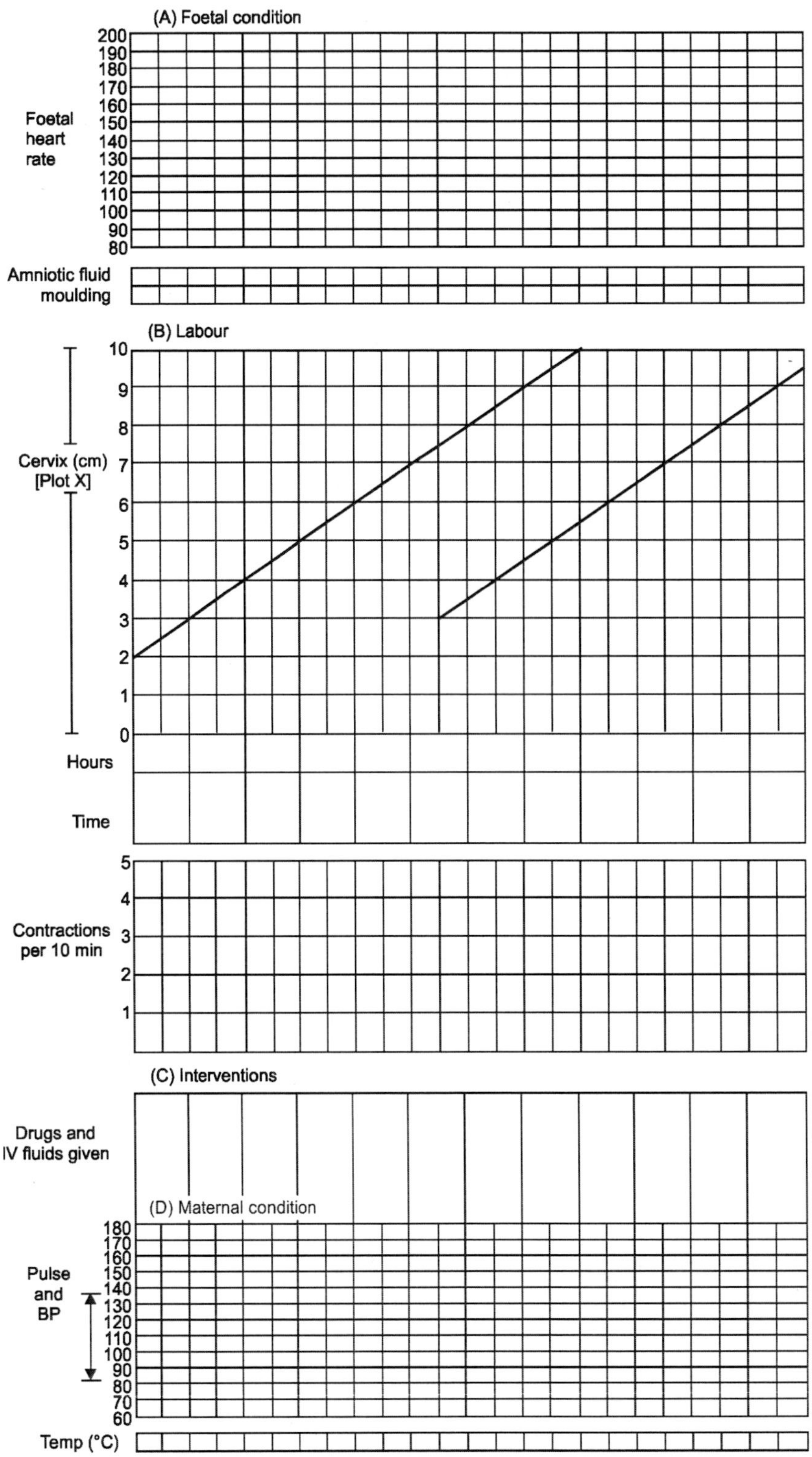

a. Delivery of Baby

Baby Born at:______________ AM/PM, Male/Female:______________________ Mode of Delivery: __________________
Condition of Baby: Active/ Nonactive/Asphyxiated ____

b. Delivery of Placenta and Membranes

Delivery at:____________________________________ AM/PM
Spontaneously/Manually Removed ____
Typeofplacenta____
PlacentaandMembranes: Complete/ Incomplete____
Weight_______________Cord Length_______________________Any Abnormality_________________________________

c. Blood Loss (Approximate Total Amount)

Before Delivery of the Placenta___________________________ ml
During Delivery of the Placenta___________________________ml
After Delivery of the Placenta_____________________________ml
Total Amount_________________________ ml

d. Perineum

Intact___________________Episiotomy___________________Laceration__________________Repair_______________

e. Medicationsgiven____

f. Length of Labour

Duration of Labour

Progress of Labour	Date	Time	Total...... Hrs..... Min.....
Contraction Started			...... Hrs..... Min.....
Full Dilatation			
Delivery of Baby			...... Hrs..... Min.....
Delivery of Placenta			...... Hrs..... Min.....
Total Time Taken for Labour			

Condition of the Mother following Delivery

Pulse_______________BP_________________ Height of Uterus______________ Vaginal Bleeding_______________________
Breastfeeding Initiated at ____

Sign of Supervisor **Sign of Student**

INTRANATAL CASE STUDY

Name:________________ Age: ________ G, P, L, A ________________
Name of the Hospital:________________ Hospital Number: ________________
Date of Admission:________________

ANTENATAL RECORD

Date of Booking:________ LMP:________ EDD:________ Gestation at 1st Visit:________

MEDICAL HISTORY

Chronic Illness:________________
Surgery:________________
Allergy:________________
Communicable Disease:________________

FAMILY HISTORY

Type of Family:
Nuclear: ________________ Number of Persons: ________________
Joint: ________________ Number of Persons: ________________

DISEASES: Chronic Illness

Hypertension:________ Diabetes:________ Genetic Diseases:________ Psychiatric Disorders:________
Others : ________________

HISTORY OF MULTIPLE BIRTHS

Number of Children :________ Girl Child:________ Boy Child________

SOCIOECONOMIC BACKGROUND

Religion:________________ Family Income:________________
Education: Husband: ________________ Wife: ________________
Occupation: Husband: ________________ Wife: ________________

MENSTRUAL HISTORY

Menarchy:________ Duration:________ Interval:________ Flow:________

MARITAL HISTORY

Age of Marriage:________________
Consanguineous: Yes/No

DIETARY PATTERN

Vegetarian: ________________ Nonvegetarian: ________________
Likes:________________ Dislikes:________________
Habits: Smoking/Drinking Alchohol/Chewing Pan/Tobacco

PAST OBSTETRICAL HISTORY

S.No	Year	Full Term	Abortion	Type of Delivery	Sex of Baby	Alive	Stillbirth	Weight	Remarks

PRESENT PREGNANCY

Admission Notes:

Admission on:____________ at:____________ Contractions Commenced:______________ at:____________________
Period of Gestation:____________________ Membranes: Intact:___________________ Ruptured on:_________________
Height of Fundus: ______________________________ Contractions ______________________________________
Presentation:___________________________________ Position:____
Engaged/Nonengaged: __________________________________ FHR: ____________________________________
Bladder :____ Bowel:_________________________________
BP:____ TPR: _______________________________________
Special Observations: ____

PRENATAL VISITS

Date of Booking	Weight	Height	Urine		BP	FHR	Weeks of Gestation	Height of Fundus	Position	Treatment
			Protein	Glucose						

EXAMINATION AND INVESTIGATIONS

Blood Group:________ Rh Factor:_________ Hb:__________ VDRL:__________ HIV:__________Others:_______________
Heart_________ Lungs____________ Breast_____________ Abdomen_______________ Perineum_________________

DELIVERY RECORD

Onset of True Labour: Date:_______________________ Time:_______________________
Time of Full Dilatation: Date:______________________ Time:_______________________
Membranes Ruptured at:_____________________ Spontaneous/Artificial: ______________ PROM:___________________

THE SIMPLIFIED PARTOGRAPH

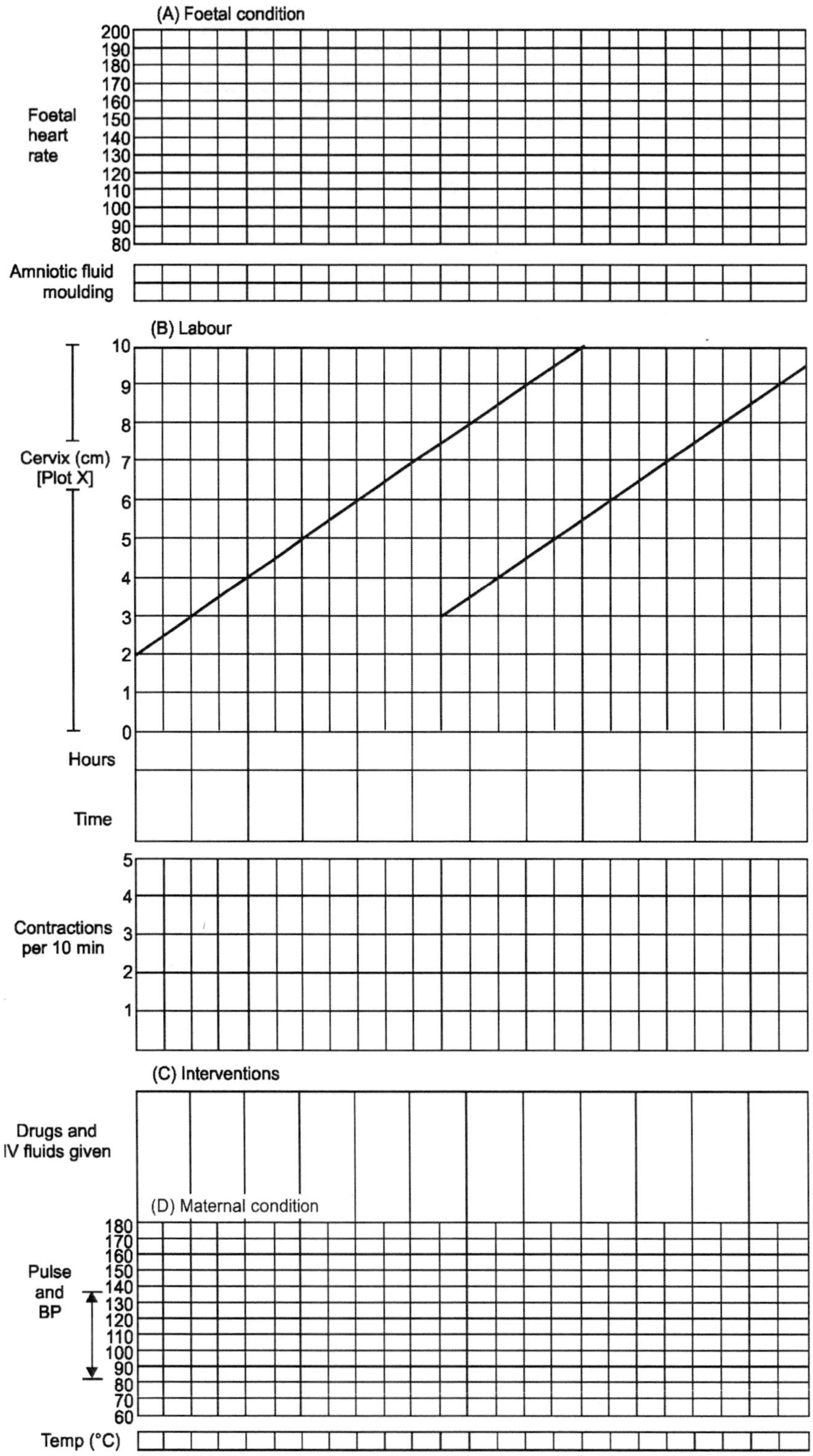

a. Delivery of Baby

Baby Born at:______________ AM/PM, Male/Female:_____________________ Mode of Delivery: ________________
Condition of Baby: Active/ Nonactive/Asphyxiated ____

b. Delivery of Placenta and Membranes

Delivery at:__________________________________ AM/PM
Spontaneously/Manually Removed ____
Typeofplacenta____
PlacentaandMembranes: Complete/Incomplete____
Weight______________Cord Length______________________Any Abnormality__________________________

c. Blood Loss (Approximate Total Amount)

Before Delivery of the Placenta_________________________ ml
During Delivery of the Placenta_________________________ml
After Delivery of the Placenta___________________________ml
Total Amount________________________ ml

d. Perineum

Intact__________________Episiotomy___________________Laceration__________________Repair_______________

e. Medicationsgiven____

f. Length of Labour

Duration of Labour

Progress of Labour	Date	Time	Total...... Hrs..... Min.....
Contraction Started			...... Hrs..... Min.....
Full Dilatation			
Delivery of Baby			...... Hrs..... Min.....
Delivery of Placenta			...... Hrs..... Min.....
Total Time Taken for Labour			

Condition of the Mother following Delivery

Pulse______________BP_________________ Height of Uterus______________ Vaginal Bleeding______________________
Breastfeeding Initiated at ____

Sign of Supervisor **Sign of Student**

INTRANATAL CASE STUDY

Name:____________________ Age: ________ G, P, L, A ____________________
Name of the Hospital:____________________ Hospital Number: ____________________
Date of Admission:____________________

ANTENATAL RECORD

Date of Booking:__________ LMP:__________ EDD:__________ Gestation at 1st Visit:__________

MEDICAL HISTORY

Chronic Illness:____________________
Surgery:____________________
Allergy:____________________
Communicable Disease:____________________

FAMILY HISTORY

Type of Family:
Nuclear: ____________________ Number of Persons: ____________________
Joint: ____________________ Number of Persons: ____________________

DISEASES: Chronic Illness

Hypertension:__________ Diabetes:__________ Genetic Diseases:__________ Psychiatric Disorders:__________
Others : ____________________

HISTORY OF MULTIPLE BIRTHS

Number of Children :__________ Girl Child:__________ Boy Child__________

SOCIOECONOMIC BACKGROUND

Religion:____________________ Family Income:____________________
Education: Husband: ____________________ Wife: ____________________
Occupation: Husband: ____________________ Wife: ____________________

MENSTRUAL HISTORY

Menarchy:__________ Duration:__________ Interval:__________ Flow:__________

MARITAL HISTORY

Age of Marriage:____________________
Consanguineous: Yes/No

DIETARY PATTERN

Vegetarian: ____________________ Nonvegetarian: ____________________
Likes:____________________ Dislikes:____________________
Habits: Smoking/Drinking Alchohol/Chewing Pan/Tobacco

PAST OBSTETRICAL HISTORY

S.No	Year	Full Term	Abortion	Type of Delivery	Sex of Baby	Alive	Stillbirth	Weight	Remarks

PRESENT PREGNANCY

Admission Notes:

Admission on:____________ at:_____________ Contractions Commenced:________________ at:__________________

Period of Gestation:_____________________ Membranes: Intact:____________________ Ruptured on:__________________

Height of Fundus: _______________________________ Contractions ____

Presentation:____________________________________ Position:____

Engaged/Nonengaged: ____________________________________ FHR: ____

Bladder :____ Bowel:_____________________________________

BP:____ TPR: ______________________________________

Special Observations: ____

PRENATAL VISITS

Date of Booking	Weight	Height	Urine		BP	FHR	Weeks of Gestation	Height of Fundus	Position	Treatment
			Protein	Glucose						

EXAMINATION AND INVESTIGATIONS

Blood Group:________ Rh Factor:_________ Hb:__________ VDRL:__________ HIV:__________Others:________________

Heart_________ Lungs____________ Breast______________ Abdomen________________ Perineum___________________

DELIVERY RECORD

Onset of True Labour: Date:_______________________ Time:________________________

Time of Full Dilatation: Date:_____________________ Time:________________________

Membranes Ruptured at:_____________________ Spontaneous/Artificial: ______________ PROM:__________________

THE SIMPLIFIED PARTOGRAPH

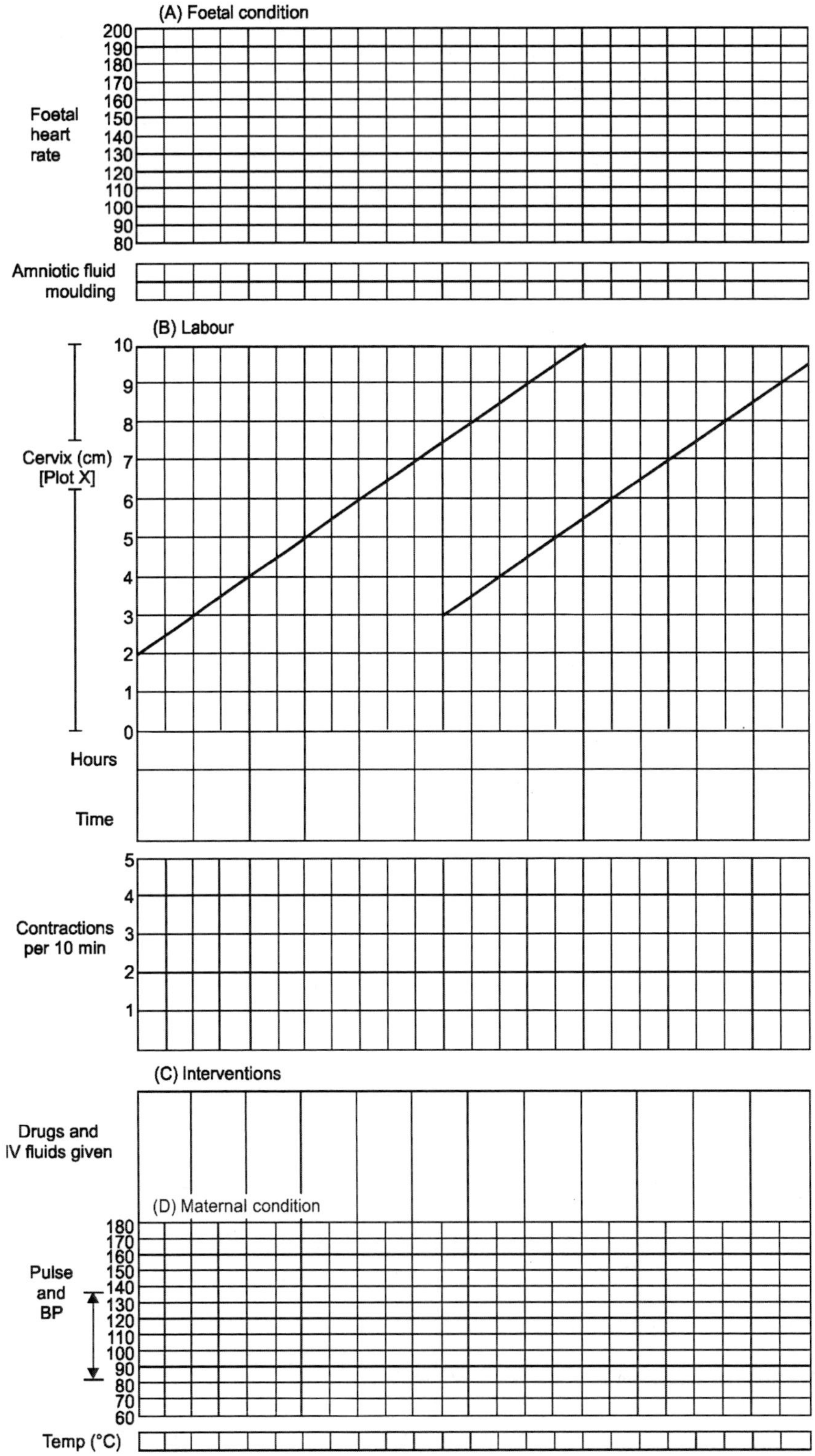

a. Delivery of Baby

Baby Born at:______________ AM/PM, Male/Female:_____________________ Mode of Delivery: _________________
Condition of Baby: Active/ Nonactive/Asphyxiated ____

b. Delivery of Placenta and Membranes

Delivery at:__________________________________ AM/PM
Spontaneously/Manually Removed ____
Typeofplacenta____
PlacentaandMembranes: Complete/ Incomplete____
Weight______________Cord Length______________________Any Abnormality___________________________

c. Blood Loss (Approximate Total Amount)

Before Delivery of the Placenta_________________________ ml
During Delivery of the Placenta_________________________ml
After Delivery of the Placenta___________________________ml
Total Amount________________________ ml

d. Perineum

Intact_________________Episiotomy___________________Laceration_________________Repair_______________

e. Medicationsgiven____

f. Length of Labour

Duration of Labour

Progress of Labour	Date	Time	Total...... Hrs..... Min.....
Contraction Started			...... Hrs..... Min.....
Full Dilatation			
Delivery of Baby			...... Hrs..... Min.....
Delivery of Placenta			...... Hrs..... Min.....
Total Time Taken for Labour			

Condition of the Mother following Delivery

Pulse______________BP_________________ Height of Uterus______________ Vaginal Bleeding______________________
Breastfeeding Initiated at ____

Sign of Supervisor **Sign of Student**

INTRANATAL CASE STUDY

Name:______________________________ Age: __________ G, P, L, A ______________________________
Name of the Hospital:____________________________ Hospital Number: ______________________________
Date of Admission:______________________________

ANTENATAL RECORD

Date of Booking:______________ LMP:__________ EDD:____________ Gestation at 1st Visit:____________

MEDICAL HISTORY

Chronic Illness:____
Surgery:____
Allergy:____
Communicable Disease:____

FAMILY HISTORY

Type of Family:
Nuclear: ____________________________ Number of Persons: ________________________
Joint: ____________________________ Number of Persons: ________________________

DISEASES: Chronic Illness

Hypertension:____________ Diabetes:__________ Genetic Diseases:__________ Psychiatric Disorders:____________
Others : ____

HISTORY OF MULTIPLE BIRTHS

Number of Children :________________ Girl Child:________________ Boy Child________________

SOCIOECONOMIC BACKGROUND

Religion:____________________________ Family Income:______________________________
Education: Husband: ____________________________ Wife: ______________________________
Occupation: Husband: ________________________ Wife: ______________________________

MENSTRUAL HISTORY

Menarchy:________________ Duration:____________ Interval:______________ Flow:____________

MARITAL HISTORY

Age of Marriage:____________________
Consanguineous: Yes/No

DIETARY PATTERN

Vegetarian: ____________________________ Nonvegetarian: ______________________________
Likes:______________________________ Dislikes:______________________________
Habits: Smoking/Drinking Alchohol/Chewing Pan/Tobacco

PAST OBSTETRICAL HISTORY

S.No	Year	Full Term	Abortion	Type of Delivery	Sex of Baby	Alive	Stillbirth	Weight	Remarks

PRESENT PREGNANCY

Admission Notes:

Admission on:____________ at:_____________ Contractions Commenced:________________ at:_________________
Period of Gestation:_____________________ Membranes: Intact:____________________ Ruptured on:_______________
Height of Fundus: _______________________________ Contractions _____________________________________
Presentation:_____________________________________ Position:____
Engaged/Nonengaged: ____________________________________ FHR: _____________________________________
Bladder :____ Bowel:______________________________
BP:____ TPR: ______________________________________
Special Observations: ____

PRENATAL VISITS

Date of Booking	Weight	Height	Urine		BP	FHR	Weeks of Gestation	Height of Fundus	Position	Treatment
			Protein	Glucose						

EXAMINATION AND INVESTIGATIONS

Blood Group:________ Rh Factor:_________ Hb:__________ VDRL:__________ HIV:__________Others:_______________
Heart_________ Lungs____________ Breast_____________ Abdomen________________ Perineum__________________

DELIVERY RECORD

Onset of True Labour: Date:________________________ Time:________________________
Time of Full Dilatation: Date:______________________ Time:________________________
Membranes Ruptured at:______________________ Spontaneous/Artificial: ______________ PROM:__________________

THE SIMPLIFIED PARTOGRAPH

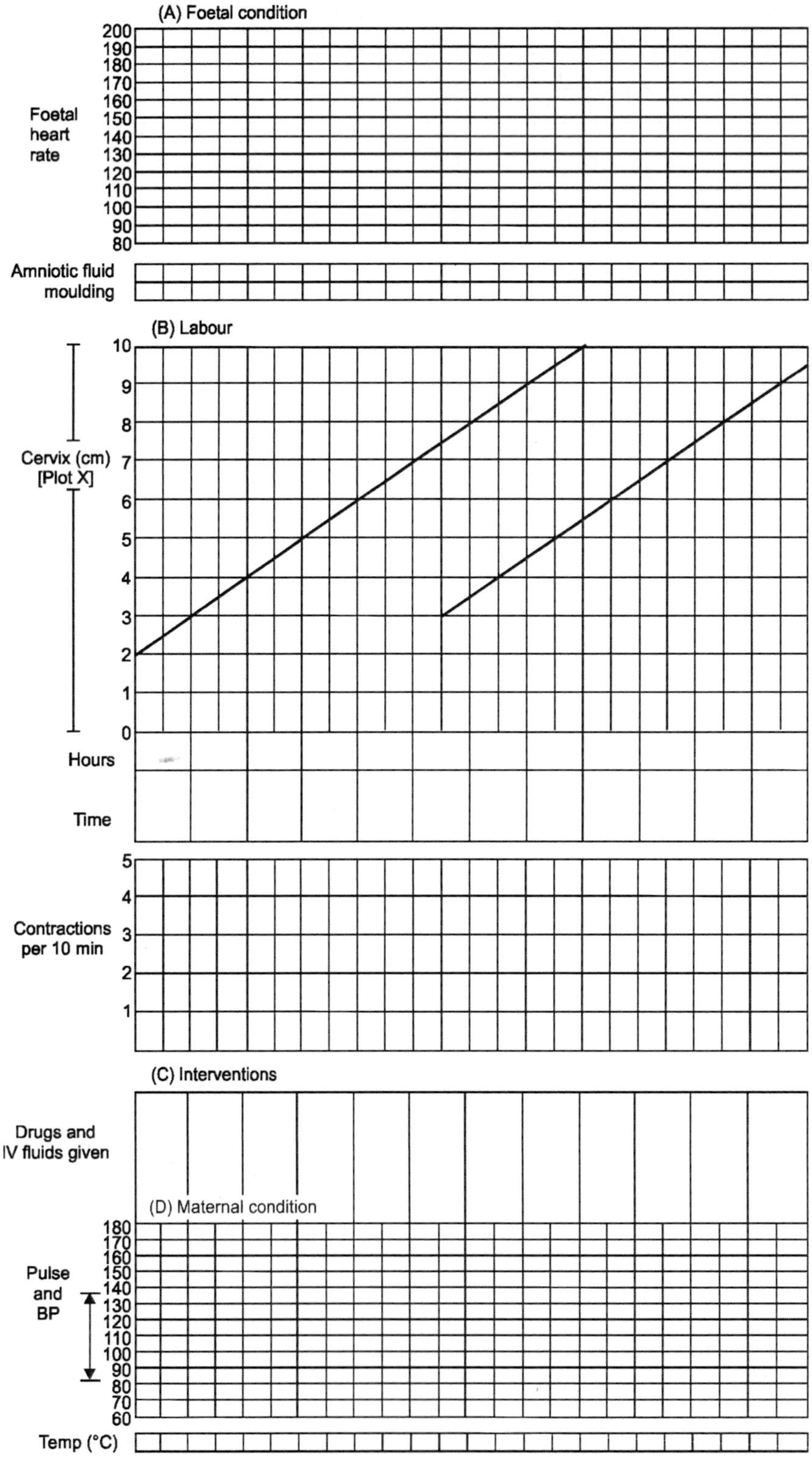

a. Delivery of Baby

Baby Born at:______________ AM/PM, Male/Female:_____________________ Mode of Delivery: __________________

Condition of Baby: Active/ Nonactive/Asphyxiated ____

b. Delivery of Placenta and Membranes

Delivery at:___________________________________ AM/PM

Spontaneously/Manually Removed ____

Typeofplacenta____

Placenta and Membranes: Complete/ Incomplete____

Weight______________ Cord Length______________________ Any Abnormality_____________________________

c. Blood Loss (Approximate Total Amount)

Before Delivery of the Placenta__________________________ ml

During Delivery of the Placenta__________________________ml

After Delivery of the Placenta____________________________ml

Total Amount________________________ ml

d. Perineum

Intact__________________ Episiotomy___________________ Laceration__________________ Repair_______________

e. Medications given____

f. Length of Labour

Duration of Labour

Progress of Labour	Date	Time	Total...... Hrs..... Min.....
Contraction Started			...... Hrs..... Min.....
Full Dilatation			
Delivery of Baby			...... Hrs..... Min.....
Delivery of Placenta			...... Hrs..... Min.....
Total Time Taken for Labour			

Condition of the Mother following Delivery

Pulse______________BP_________________ Height of Uterus______________ Vaginal Bleeding______________________

Breastfeeding Initiated at ____

Sign of Supervisor **Sign of Student**

INTRANATAL CASE STUDY

Name:____________________ Age: __________ G, P, L, A ____________________
Name of the Hospital:____________________ Hospital Number: ____________________
Date of Admission:____________________

ANTENATAL RECORD

Date of Booking:__________ LMP:__________ EDD:__________ Gestation at 1st Visit:__________

MEDICAL HISTORY

Chronic Illness:____________________
Surgery:____________________
Allergy:____________________
Communicable Disease:____________________

FAMILY HISTORY

Type of Family:
Nuclear: ____________________ Number of Persons: ____________________
Joint: ____________________ Number of Persons: ____________________

DISEASES: Chronic Illness

Hypertension:__________ Diabetes:__________ Genetic Diseases:__________ Psychiatric Disorders:__________
Others : ____________________

HISTORY OF MULTIPLE BIRTHS

Number of Children :__________ Girl Child:__________ Boy Child__________

SOCIOECONOMIC BACKGROUND

Religion:____________________ Family Income:____________________
Education: Husband: ____________________ Wife: ____________________
Occupation: Husband: ____________________ Wife: ____________________

MENSTRUAL HISTORY

Menarchy:__________ Duration:__________ Interval:__________ Flow:__________

MARITAL HISTORY

Age of Marriage:____________________
Consanguineous: Yes/No

DIETARY PATTERN

Vegetarian: ____________________ Nonvegetarian: ____________________
Likes:____________________ Dislikes:____________________
Habits: Smoking/Drinking Alchohol/Chewing Pan/Tobacco

PAST OBSTETRICAL HISTORY

S.No	Year	Full Term	Abortion	Type of Delivery	Sex of Baby	Alive	Stillbirth	Weight	Remarks

PRESENT PREGNANCY

Admission Notes:

Admission on:______________ at: ________________ Contractions Commenced:___________________ at:_________________________

Period of Gestation:________________________ Membranes: Intact:_______________________ Ruptured on:____________________

Height of Fundus: _____________________________________ Contractions ____

Presentation:____ Position:____

Engaged/Nonengaged: ____ FHR: ____

Bladder :____ Bowel:____

BP:____ TPR: ____

Special Observations: ____

PRENATAL VISITS

Date of Booking	Weight	Height	Urine		BP	FHR	Weeks of Gestation	Height of Fundus	Position	Treatment
			Protein	Glucose						

EXAMINATION AND INVESTIGATIONS

Blood Group:_________ Rh Factor:__________ Hb:___________ VDRL:___________ HIV:___________Others:_________________

Heart__________ Lungs_____________ Breast_______________ Abdomen_________________ Perineum____________________

DELIVERY RECORD

Onset of True Labour: Date:____________________________ Time:___________________________

Time of Full Dilatation: Date:__________________________ Time:___________________________

Membranes Ruptured at:_________________________ Spontaneous/Artificial: _______________ PROM:____________________

THE SIMPLIFIED PARTOGRAPH

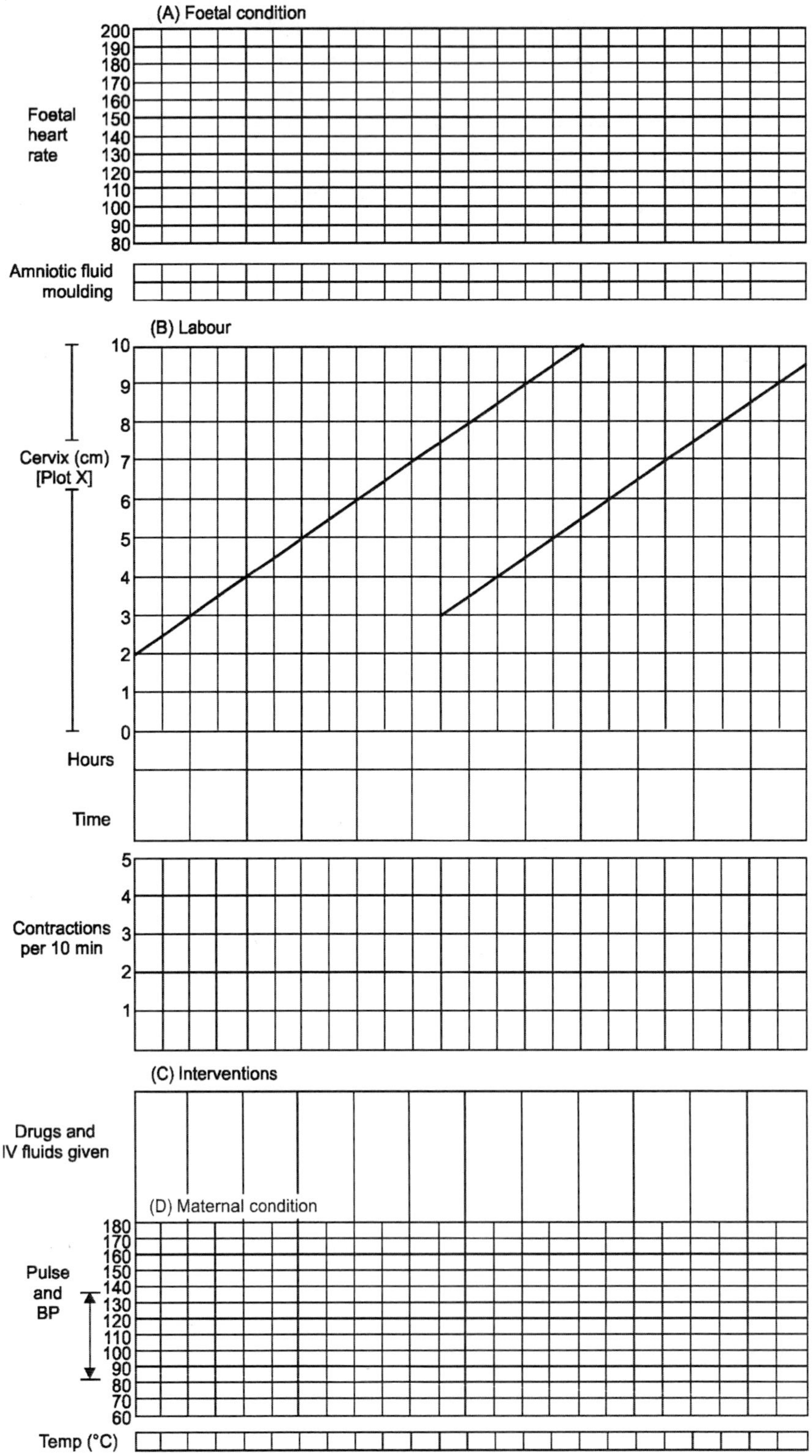

a. Delivery of Baby

Baby Born at:______________ AM/PM, Male/Female:_____________________ Mode of Delivery: ________________
Condition of Baby: Active/ Nonactive/Asphyxiated ____

b. Delivery of Placenta and Membranes

Delivery at:_______________________________ AM/PM
Spontaneously/Manually Removed ____
Typeofplacenta____
PlacentaandMembranes: Complete/Incomplete____
Weight______________Cord Length_____________________Any Abnormality________________________

c. Blood Loss (Approximate Total Amount)

Before Delivery of the Placenta_________________________ ml
During Delivery of the Placenta_________________________ml
After Delivery of the Placenta___________________________ml
Total Amount________________________ ml

d. Perineum

Intact_________________Episiotomy__________________Laceration_________________Repair______________

e. Medicationsgiven____

f. Length of Labour

Duration of Labour

Progress of Labour	Date	Time	Total...... Hrs..... Min.....
Contraction Started			...... Hrs..... Min.....
Full Dilatation			
Delivery of Baby			...... Hrs..... Min.....
Delivery of Placenta			...... Hrs..... Min.....
Total Time Taken for Labour			

Condition of the Mother following Delivery

Pulse______________BP_________________ Height of Uterus______________ Vaginal Bleeding_____________________
Breastfeeding Initiated at ____

Sign of Supervisor **Sign of Student**

INTRANATAL CASE STUDY

Name:________________ Age: ________ G, P, L, A ________________
Name of the Hospital:________________ Hospital Number: ________________
Date of Admission:________________

ANTENATAL RECORD

Date of Booking:________ LMP:________ EDD:________ Gestation at 1st Visit:________

MEDICAL HISTORY

Chronic Illness:________________
Surgery:________________
Allergy:________________
Communicable Disease:________________

FAMILY HISTORY

Type of Family:
Nuclear: ________________ Number of Persons: ________________
Joint: ________________ Number of Persons: ________________

DISEASES: Chronic Illness

Hypertension:________ Diabetes:________ Genetic Diseases:________ Psychiatric Disorders:________
Others : ________________

HISTORY OF MULTIPLE BIRTHS

Number of Children :________ Girl Child:________ Boy Child________

SOCIOECONOMIC BACKGROUND

Religion:________________ Family Income:________________
Education: Husband: ________________ Wife: ________________
Occupation: Husband: ________________ Wife: ________________

MENSTRUAL HISTORY

Menarchy:________ Duration:________ Interval:________ Flow:________

MARITAL HISTORY

Age of Marriage:________________
Consanguineous: Yes/No

DIETARY PATTERN

Vegetarian: ________________ Nonvegetarian: ________________
Likes:________________ Dislikes:________________
Habits: Smoking/Drinking Alchohol/Chewing Pan/Tobacco

PAST OBSTETRICAL HISTORY

S.No	Year	Full Term	Abortion	Type of Delivery	Sex of Baby	Alive	Stillbirth	Weight	Remarks

PRESENT PREGNANCY

Admission Notes:

Admission on:____________ at:____________ Contractions Commenced:______________ at:__________________

Period of Gestation:____________________ Membranes: Intact:____________________ Ruptured on:________________

Height of Fundus: ______________________________ Contractions ____

Presentation:____________________________________ Position:____

Engaged/Nonengaged: ___________________________________ FHR: ____

Bladder :____ Bowel:____

BP:____ TPR: ____

Special Observations: ____

PRENATAL VISITS

Date of Booking	Weight	Height	Urine		BP	FHR	Weeks of Gestation	Height of Fundus	Position	Treatment
			Protein	Glucose						

EXAMINATION AND INVESTIGATIONS

Blood Group:________ Rh Factor:_________ Hb:__________ VDRL:__________ HIV:__________Others:________________

Heart_________ Lungs____________ Breast______________ Abdomen________________ Perineum__________________

DELIVERY RECORD

Onset of True Labour: Date:_______________________ Time:______________________

Time of Full Dilatation: Date:_____________________ Time:______________________

Membranes Ruptured at:_____________________ Spontaneous/Artificial: ______________ PROM:__________________

THE SIMPLIFIED PARTOGRAPH

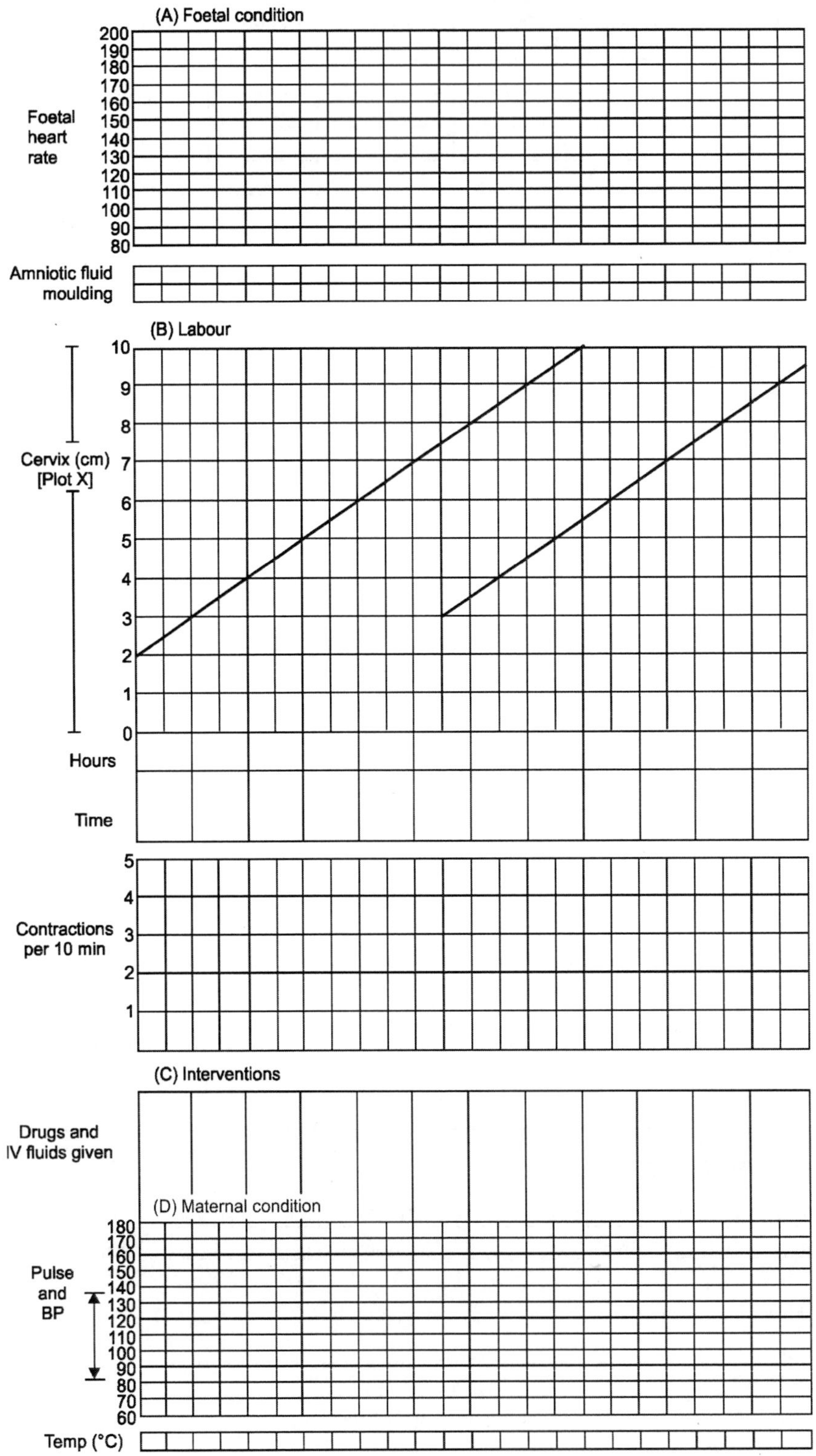

a. Delivery of Baby

Baby Born at:______________ AM/PM, Male/Female:_____________________ Mode of Delivery: __________________
Condition of Baby: Active/ Nonactive/Asphyxiated ____

b. Delivery of Placenta and Membranes

Delivery at:___________________________________ AM/PM
Spontaneously/Manually Removed ____
Typeofplacenta____
PlacentaandMembranes: Complete/Incomplete____
Weight______________Cord Length______________________Any Abnormality___________________________________

c. Blood Loss (Approximate Total Amount)

Before Delivery of the Placenta__________________________ ml
During Delivery of the Placenta__________________________ml
After Delivery of the Placenta___________________________ml
Total Amount_________________________ ml

d. Perineum

Intact__________________Episiotomy___________________Laceration__________________Repair_______________

e. Medicationsgiven____

f. Length of Labour

Duration of Labour

Progress of Labour	Date	Time	Total...... Hrs..... Min.....
Contraction Started			...... Hrs..... Min.....
Full Dilatation			
Delivery of Baby			...... Hrs..... Min.....
Delivery of Placenta			...... Hrs..... Min.....
Total Time Taken for Labour			

Condition of the Mother following Delivery

Pulse______________BP_________________ Height of Uterus______________ Vaginal Bleeding______________________
Breastfeeding Initiated at ____

Sign of Supervisor **Sign of Student**

POSTNATAL EXAMINATION

POSTNATAL CARE

Name:____________________ Age:________ G, P, L, A ____________________
Name of the Hospital:____________________ Hospital Number: ____________________
Date of Delivery:____________________ Date of Discharge:____________________
Date of Registration:____________________ LMP: ________ EDD: ____________________
Prenatal Record:____________________ Gestation at 1st visit: ____________________

MEDICAL HISTORY

Chronic Illness:____________________
Surgery:____________________
Allergy:____________________
Communicable Disease:____________________

FAMILY HISTORY

Type of Family:
Nuclear:____________________ Number of Persons:____________________
Joint:____________________ Number of Persons:____________________

HISTORY OF MULTIPLE BIRTHS

Number of Children:____________________ Girl Child:__________ Boy Child____________________

SOCIOECONOMIC BACKGROUND

Religion:____________________ Family Income:____________________
Education: Husband:____________________ Wife: ____________________
Occupation: Husband: ____________________ Wife: ____________________

DISEASES: Chronic Illness: __________ Genetic Disorder: __________ Psychiatric Disorder:__________

MENSTRUAL HISTORY

Menarchy:________________Duration:____________Interval:______________Flow:________

MARITAL HISTORY

Age of marriage:____________________ Year of Marriage: ____________________
Consanguineous: Yes/No

DIETARY PATTERN

Vegetarian:________________ Nonvegetarian: ____________________
Likes: ____________________ Dislikes: ____________________
Habits: Smoking/Drinking Alchohol/Chewing pan/Tobacco

PAST OBSTETRICAL HISTORY

S.No	Year	Full Term	Abortion	Type of Delivery	Sex of Baby	Alive	Stillbirth	Weight	Remarks

PRESENT PREGNANCY

Admission Notes:

Admission on:____________ at:____________ Contractions Commenced:____________ at:____________

Period of Gestation:____________ Membranes: Intact:____________ Ruptured on:____________

Involution of Uterus:____________ Contractions____________

Presentation:____________ Position:____________

Engaged/Nonengaged:____________ FHR: ____________

Bladder:____________ Bowel: ____________

BP:____________ TPR: ____________

Special Observations:____________

PRENATAL VISITS

Date of Booking	Weight	Height	Urine		BP	FHR	Weeks of Gestation	Height of Fundus	Position	Treatment
			Protein	Glucose						

GENERAL CONDITION

BP:________ TPR:________________________ Urine: Sp. gavity________________ Reaction:______________
Protein:______________________ Glucose:____________________ Acetone:______________________________

EXAMINATION AND INVESTIGATIONS

Blood Group:________ Rh Factor:________ Hb:________ VDRL:________ HIV:________Others:______________
Heart________ Lungs__________ Breast___________ Abdomen______________ Perineum______________

DELIVERY RECORD

Onset of True Labour: Date:______________ Time:_________________
Time of Full Dilatation: Date:____________________ Time:______________________
Membranes Ruptured at:____________________ Spontaneous/Artificial: ______________ PROM:________________

a. Delivery of Baby

Baby Born at:________________ AM/PM, Male/Female:____________ Mode of Delivery:________________
Condition of Baby: Active/Nonactive/Asphyxiated _______________ Apgar Score ______________________
Treatment: ____

b. Delivery of Placenta and Membranes

Delivery at:_______________ AM/PM
Spontaneously/Manually removed____
Type of placenta____
Placenta and membranes: Complete/Incomplete_______________________________________
Weight _____________ Cord Length__________________ Any Abnormality__________________________
Total Blood Loss:____

c. Perineum

Intact__________ Episiotomy_______________ Laceration_______________________ Repair________________
Medications Given ____
____
____

d. Length of Labour

Mode of Delivery: ____

DURATION OF LABOUR

Progress of Labour	Date	Time	Total...... Hrs..... Min.....
Contraction Started			...... Hrs..... Min.....
Full Dilatation			
Delivery of Baby			...... Hrs..... Min.....
Delivery of Placenta			...... Hrs..... Min.....
Total Time Taken for Labour			

e. Condition of the Mother following Delivery

Pulse: ____________________BP:____________________ Uterus: Hard/Soft Vaginal bleeding: ____________________
Breastfeeding initiated at: ____
Perineum Scar: Healthy/Not healthy

CLINICAL CHART OF BABY

Date: Temperature:																	
°F	°C																
104.0	40																
103.1	39.5																
102.2	39																
101.3	38.5																
100.4	38																
99.5	37.5																
98.6	37																
97.7	36.5																
96.8	36																
Heart Rate																	
Respiration																	
Urine																	
Stool																	
Vomit																	
Jaundice																	
Weight																	
Remarks																	

CLINICAL CHART OF PUERPERIUM

Date: Temperature:																	
°F	°C																
104.0	40																
103.1	39.5																
102.2	39																
101.3	38.5																
100.4	38																
99.5	37.5																
98.6	37																
97.7	36.5																
96.8	36																
95.9	35.5																
Respiration																	
BP																	
Lochia																	
Urine																	
Motion																	
Fundus in cm																	

Sign of Supervisor **Sign of Student**

POSTNATAL CARE

Name:____________________ Age:__________ G, P, L, A ____________________
Name of the Hospital:____________________ Hospital Number: ____________________
Date of Delivery:____________________ Date of Discharge:____________________
Date of Registration:____________________ LMP: __________ EDD: ____________________
Prenatal Record:____________________ Gestation at 1st visit: ____________________

MEDICAL HISTORY

Chronic Illness:____________________
Surgery:____________________
Allergy:____________________
Communicable Disease:____________________

FAMILY HISTORY

Type of Family:
Nuclear:____________________ Number of Persons:____________________
Joint:____________________ Number of Persons:____________________

HISTORY OF MULTIPLE BIRTHS

Number of Children:__________ Girl Child:__________ Boy Child__________

SOCIOECONOMIC BACKGROUND

Religion:____________________ Family Income:____________________
Education: Husband:____________________ Wife: ____________________
Occupation: Husband: ____________________ Wife: ____________________

DISEASES: Chronic Illness: __________ Genetic Disorder: __________ Psychiatric Disorder:__________

MENSTRUAL HISTORY

Menarchy:__________Duration:__________Interval:__________Flow:__________

MARITAL HISTORY

Age of marriage:____________________ Year of Marriage: ____________________
Consanguineous: Yes/No

DIETARY PATTERN

Vegetarian:__________ Nonvegetarian: __________
Likes: __________ Dislikes: __________
Habits: Smoking/Drinking Alchohol/Chewing pan/Tobacco

PAST OBSTETRICAL HISTORY

S.No	Year	Full Term	Abortion	Type of Delivery	Sex of Baby	Alive	Stillbirth	Weight	Remarks

PRESENT PREGNANCY

Admission Notes:

Admission on:__________ at:__________ Contractions Commenced:__________ at:__________

Period of Gestation:__________ Membranes: Intact:__________ Ruptured on:__________

Involution of Uterus:__________ Contractions__________

Presentation:__________ Position:__________

Engaged/Nonengaged:__________ FHR:__________

Bladder:__________ Bowel:__________

BP:__________ TPR:__________

Special Observations:__________

PRENATAL VISITS

Date of Booking	Weight	Height	Urine		BP	FHR	Weeks of Gestation	Height of Fundus	Position	Treatment
			Protein	Glucose						

GENERAL CONDITION

BP:________ TPR:__________________________ Urine: Sp. gavity__________________ Reaction:______________
Protein:_______________________ Glucose:_____________________ Acetone:________________________________

EXAMINATION AND INVESTIGATIONS

Blood Group:________ Rh Factor:_________ Hb:__________ VDRL:__________ HIV:__________Others:_______________
Heart_________ Lungs____________ Breast_____________ Abdomen_________________ Perineum___________________

DELIVERY RECORD

Onset of True Labour: Date:_______________ Time:___________________
Time of Full Dilatation: Date:______________________ Time:________________________
Membranes Ruptured at:_____________________ Spontaneous/Artificial: ______________ PROM:__________________

a. Delivery of Baby

Baby Born at:_________________ AM/PM, Male/Female:_____________ Mode of Delivery:______________________
Condition of Baby: Active/Nonactive/Asphyxiated _______________ Apgar Score _____________________________
Treatment: ____

b. Delivery of Placenta and Membranes

Delivery at:________________ AM/PM
Spontaneously/Manually removed____
Type of placenta____
Placenta and membranes: Complete/Incomplete____
Weight _____________ Cord Length___________________ Any Abnormality____________________________________
Total Blood Loss:____

c. Perineum

Intact___________ Episiotomy________________ Laceration_________________________ Repair__________________
Medications Given ____
____
____

d. Length of Labour

Mode of Delivery: ____

DURATION OF LABOUR

Progress of Labour	Date	Time	Total...... Hrs..... Min.....
Contraction Started			...... Hrs..... Min.....
Full Dilatation			
Delivery of Baby			...... Hrs..... Min.....
Delivery of Placenta			...... Hrs..... Min.....
Total Time Taken for Labour			

e. Condition of the Mother following Delivery

Pulse: ____________________BP:____________________ Uterus: Hard/Soft Vaginal bleeding: ____________________
Breastfeeding initiated at: ____
Perineum Scar: Healthy/Not healthy

CLINICAL CHART OF BABY

Date: Temperature:																	
°F	°C																
104.0	40																
103.1	39.5																
102.2	39																
101.3	38.5																
100.4	38																
99.5	37.5																
98.6	37																
97.7	36.5																
96.8	36																
Heart Rate																	
Respiration																	
Urine																	
Stool																	
Vomit																	
Jaundice																	
Weight																	
Remarks																	

CLINICAL CHART OF PUERPERIUM

Date: Temperature:																	
°F	**°C**																
104.0	40																
103.1	39.5																
102.2	39																
101.3	38.5																
100.4	38																
99.5	37.5																
98.6	37																
97.7	36.5																
96.8	36																
95.9	35.5																
Respiration																	
BP																	
Lochia																	
Urine																	
Motion																	
Fundus in cm																	

Sign of Supervisor **Sign of Student**

POSTNATAL CARE

Name:__________ Age:__________ G, P, L, A __________
Name of the Hospital:__________ Hospital Number: __________
Date of Delivery:__________ Date of Discharge:__________
Date of Registration:__________ LMP: __________ EDD: __________
Prenatal Record:__________ Gestation at 1st visit: __________

MEDICAL HISTORY

Chronic Illness:__________
Surgery:__________
Allergy:__________
Communicable Disease:__________

FAMILY HISTORY

Type of Family:
Nuclear:__________ Number of Persons:__________
Joint:__________ Number of Persons:__________

HISTORY OF MULTIPLE BIRTHS

Number of Children:__________ Girl Child:__________ Boy Child__________

SOCIOECONOMIC BACKGROUND

Religion:__________ Family Income:__________
Education: Husband:__________ Wife: __________
Occupation: Husband: __________ Wife: __________

DISEASES: Chronic Illness: __________ Genetic Disorder: __________ Psychiatric Disorder:__________

MENSTRUAL HISTORY

Menarchy:__________ Duration:__________ Interval:__________ Flow:__________

MARITAL HISTORY

Age of marriage:__________ Year of Marriage: __________
Consanguineous: Yes/No

DIETARY PATTERN

Vegetarian:__________ Nonvegetarian: __________
Likes: __________ Dislikes: __________
Habits: Smoking/Drinking Alchohol/Chewing pan/Tobacco

PAST OBSTETRICAL HISTORY

S.No	Year	Full Term	Abortion	Type of Delivery	Sex of Baby	Alive	Stillbirth	Weight	Remarks

PRESENT PREGNANCY

Admission Notes:

Admission on:____________ at: ____________ Contractions Commenced:____________ at:____________

Period of Gestation:____________ Membranes: Intact:____________ Ruptured on:____________

Involution of Uterus:____________ Contractions____________

Presentation:____________ Position:____________

Engaged/Nonengaged:____________ FHR: ____________

Bladder:____________ Bowel: ____________

BP:____________ TPR: ____________

Special Observations:____________

PRENATAL VISITS

Date of Booking	Weight	Height	Urine		BP	FHR	Weeks of Gestation	Height of Fundus	Position	Treatment
			Protein	Glucose						

GENERAL CONDITION

BP:________ TPR:__________________________ Urine: Sp. gavity__________________ Reaction:______________
Protein:________________________ Glucose:____________________ Acetone:______________________________________

EXAMINATION AND INVESTIGATIONS

Blood Group:________ Rh Factor:_________ Hb:__________ VDRL:__________ HIV:__________Others:________________
Heart_________ Lungs____________ Breast_____________ Abdomen________________ Perineum___________________

DELIVERY RECORD

Onset of True Labour: Date:_______________ Time:__________________
Time of Full Dilatation: Date:______________________ Time:_______________________
Membranes Ruptured at:______________________ Spontaneous/Artificial: ______________ PROM:__________________

a. Delivery of Baby

Baby Born at:__________________ AM/PM, Male/Female:_____________ Mode of Delivery:_______________________
Condition of Baby: Active/Nonactive/Asphyxiated _______________ Apgar Score _____________________________
Treatment: ____

b. Delivery of Placenta and Membranes

Delivery at:________________ AM/PM
Spontaneously/Manually removed____
Type of placenta____
Placenta and membranes: Complete/Incomplete____
Weight _____________ Cord Length___________________ Any Abnormality_____________________________
Total Blood Loss:____

c. Perineum

Intact___________ Episiotomy________________ Laceration_________________________ Repair_________________
Medications Given ____
____
____

d. Length of Labour

Mode of Delivery: ____

DURATION OF LABOUR

Progress of Labour	Date	Time	Total...... Hrs..... Min.....
Contraction Started			...... Hrs..... Min.....
Full Dilatation			
Delivery of Baby			...... Hrs..... Min.....
Delivery of Placenta			...... Hrs..... Min.....
Total Time Taken for Labour			

e. Condition of the Mother following Delivery

Pulse: ________________BP:________________ Uterus: Hard/Soft Vaginal bleeding: ________________

Breastfeeding initiated at: ____

Perineum Scar: Healthy/Not healthy

CLINICAL CHART OF BABY

Date: Temperature:																	
°F	**°C**																
104.0	40																
103.1	39.5																
102.2	39																
101.3	38.5																
100.4	38																
99.5	37.5																
98.6	37																
97.7	36.5																
96.8	36																
Heart Rate																	
Respiration																	
Urine																	
Stool																	
Vomit																	
Jaundice																	
Weight																	
Remarks																	

CLINICAL CHART OF PUERPERIUM

Date: Temperature:																	
°F	**°C**																
104.0	40																
103.1	39.5																
102.2	39																
101.3	38.5																
100.4	38																
99.5	37.5																
98.6	37																
97.7	36.5																
96.8	36																
95.9	35.5																
Respiration																	
BP																	
Lochia																	
Urine																	
Motion																	
Fundus in cm																	

Sign of Supervisor **Sign of Student**

POSTNATAL CARE

Name:__________ Age:__________ G, P, L, A __________
Name of the Hospital:__________ Hospital Number: __________
Date of Delivery:__________ Date of Discharge:__________
Date of Registration:__________ LMP: __________ EDD: __________
Prenatal Record:__________ Gestation at 1st visit: __________

MEDICAL HISTORY

Chronic Illness:__________
Surgery:__________
Allergy:__________
Communicable Disease:__________

FAMILY HISTORY

Type of Family:
Nuclear:__________ Number of Persons:__________
Joint:__________ Number of Persons:__________

HISTORY OF MULTIPLE BIRTHS

Number of Children:__________ Girl Child:__________ Boy Child__________

SOCIOECONOMIC BACKGROUND

Religion:__________ Family Income:__________
Education: Husband:__________ Wife: __________
Occupation: Husband: __________ Wife: __________

DISEASES: Chronic Illness: __________ Genetic Disorder: __________ Psychiatric Disorder:__________

MENSTRUAL HISTORY

Menarchy:__________Duration:__________Interval:__________Flow:__________

MARITAL HISTORY

Age of marriage:__________ Year of Marriage: __________
Consanguineous: Yes/No

DIETARY PATTERN

Vegetarian:__________ Nonvegetarian: __________
Likes: __________ Dislikes: __________
Habits: Smoking/Drinking Alchohol/Chewing pan/Tobacco

PAST OBSTETRICAL HISTORY

S.No	Year	Full Term	Abortion	Type of Delivery	Sex of Baby	Alive	Stillbirth	Weight	Remarks

PRESENT PREGNANCY

Admission Notes:

Admission on:____________ at:____________ Contractions Commenced:____________ at:____________

Period of Gestation:____________ Membranes: Intact:____________ Ruptured on:____________

Involution of Uterus:____________ Contractions____________

Presentation:____________ Position:____________

Engaged/Nonengaged:____________ FHR:____________

Bladder:____________ Bowel:____________

BP:____________ TPR:____________

Special Observations:____________

PRENATAL VISITS

Date of Booking	Weight	Height	Urine		BP	FHR	Weeks of Gestation	Height of Fundus	Position	Treatment
			Protein	Glucose						

GENERAL CONDITION

BP:________ TPR:__________________________ Urine: Sp. gavity__________________ Reaction:______________
Protein:________________________ Glucose:____________________ Acetone:____

EXAMINATION AND INVESTIGATIONS

Blood Group:________ Rh Factor:_________ Hb:__________ VDRL:__________ HIV:__________Others:________________
Heart_________ Lungs____________ Breast_____________ Abdomen________________ Perineum__________________

DELIVERY RECORD

Onset of True Labour: Date:_______________ Time:__________________
Time of Full Dilatation: Date:______________________ Time:________________________
Membranes Ruptured at:______________________ Spontaneous/Artificial: ______________ PROM:____________________

a. Delivery of Baby

Baby Born at:__________________ AM/PM, Male/Female:______________ Mode of Delivery:_______________________
Condition of Baby: Active/Nonactive/Asphyxiated ________________ Apgar Score ______________________________
Treatment: ____

b. Delivery of Placenta and Membranes

Delivery at:________________ AM/PM
Spontaneously/Manually removed____
Type of placenta____
Placenta and membranes: Complete/Incomplete____
Weight _____________ Cord Length__________________ Any Abnormality___________________________
Total Blood Loss:____

c. Perineum

Intact___________ Episiotomy________________ Laceration__________________________ Repair__________________
Medications Given ____
____
____

d. Length of Labour

Mode of Delivery: ____

DURATION OF LABOUR

Progress of Labour	Date	Time	Total...... Hrs..... Min.....
Contraction Started			...... Hrs..... Min.....
Full Dilatation			
Delivery of Baby			...... Hrs..... Min.....
Delivery of Placenta			...... Hrs..... Min.....
Total Time Taken for Labour			

e. Condition of the Mother following Delivery

Pulse: ____________________BP:____________________ Uterus: Hard/Soft Vaginal bleeding: ____________________

Breastfeeding initiated at: ____

Perineum Scar: Healthy/Not healthy

CLINICAL CHART OF BABY

Date: Temperature:																
°F	°C															
104.0	40															
103.1	39.5															
102.2	39															
101.3	38.5															
100.4	38															
99.5	37.5															
98.6	37															
97.7	36.5															
96.8	36															
Heart Rate																
Respiration																
Urine																
Stool																
Vomit																
Jaundice																
Weight																
Remarks																

CLINICAL CHART OF PUERPERIUM

Date: Temperature:																
°F	°C															
104.0	40															
103.1	39.5															
102.2	39															
101.3	38.5															
100.4	38															
99.5	37.5															
98.6	37															
97.7	36.5															
96.8	36															
95.9	35.5															
Respiration																
BP																
Lochia																
Urine																
Motion																
Fundus in cm																

Sign of Supervisor **Sign of Student**

POSTNATAL CARE

Name:____________________ Age:________ G, P, L, A ____________________
Name of the Hospital:____________________ Hospital Number: ____________________
Date of Delivery:____________________ Date of Discharge:____________________
Date of Registration:____________________ LMP: ________ EDD: ____________________
Prenatal Record:____________________ Gestation at 1st visit: ____________________

MEDICAL HISTORY

Chronic Illness:____________________
Surgery:____________________
Allergy:____________________
Communicable Disease:____________________

FAMILY HISTORY

Type of Family:
Nuclear:____________________ Number of Persons:____________________
Joint:____________________ Number of Persons:____________________

HISTORY OF MULTIPLE BIRTHS

Number of Children:____________________ Girl Child:____________ Boy Child____________________

SOCIOECONOMIC BACKGROUND

Religion:____________________ Family Income:____________________
Education: Husband:____________________ Wife: ____________________
Occupation: Husband: ____________________ Wife: ____________________

DISEASES: Chronic Illness: ____________ Genetic Disorder: ____________ Psychiatric Disorder:____________

MENSTRUAL HISTORY

Menarchy:____________Duration:____________Interval:____________Flow:____________

MARITAL HISTORY

Age of marriage:____________________ Year of Marriage: ____________________
Consanguineous: Yes/No

DIETARY PATTERN

Vegetarian:____________________ Nonvegetarian: ____________________
Likes: ____________________ Dislikes: ____________________
Habits: Smoking/Drinking Alchohol/Chewing pan/Tobacco

PAST OBSTETRICAL HISTORY

S.No	Year	Full Term	Abortion	Type of Delivery	Sex of Baby	Alive	Stillbirth	Weight	Remarks

PRESENT PREGNANCY

Admission Notes:

Admission on:____________ at:_____________ Contractions Commenced:_____________ at:__________________________

Period of Gestation:_____________________ Membranes: Intact:_________________ Ruptured on:____________________

Involution of Uterus:________________________________ Contractions______________________________________

Presentation:_____________________________________ Position:____

Engaged/Nonengaged:______________________________ FHR: ____

Bladder:____ Bowel: _______________________________________

BP:____ TPR: ____

Special Observations:____

PRENATAL VISITS

Date of Booking	Weight	Height	Urine		BP	FHR	Weeks of Gestation	Height of Fundus	Position	Treatment
			Protein	Glucose						

GENERAL CONDITION

BP:________ TPR:__________________________ Urine: Sp. gavity__________________ Reaction:______________
Protein:________________________ Glucose:____________________ Acetone:__________________________________

EXAMINATION AND INVESTIGATIONS

Blood Group:________ Rh Factor:________ Hb:__________ VDRL:__________ HIV:__________Others:________________
Heart_________ Lungs____________ Breast_____________ Abdomen________________ Perineum__________________

DELIVERY RECORD

Onset of True Labour: Date:_______________ Time:_________________
Time of Full Dilatation: Date:______________________ Time:_______________________
Membranes Ruptured at:_____________________ Spontaneous/Artificial: ______________ PROM:__________________

a. Delivery of Baby

Baby Born at:__________________ AM/PM, Male/Female:____________ Mode of Delivery:________________________
Condition of Baby: Active/Nonactive/Asphyxiated _______________ Apgar Score ______________________________
Treatment: ____

b. Delivery of Placenta and Membranes

Delivery at:________________ AM/PM
Spontaneously/Manually removed____
Type of placenta____
Placenta and membranes: Complete/Incomplete____
Weight _____________ Cord Length___________________ Any Abnormality___________________________________
Total Blood Loss:____

c. Perineum

Intact___________ Episiotomy________________ Laceration_________________________ Repair__________________
Medications Given ____
____
____

d. Length of Labour

Mode of Delivery: ____

DURATION OF LABOUR

Progress of Labour	Date	Time	Total...... Hrs..... Min.....
Contraction Started			...... Hrs..... Min.....
Full Dilatation			
Delivery of Baby			...... Hrs..... Min.....
Delivery of Placenta			...... Hrs..... Min.....
Total Time Taken for Labour			

e. Condition of the Mother following Delivery

Pulse: ____________________ BP: ____________________ Uterus: Hard/Soft Vaginal bleeding: ____________________

Breastfeeding initiated at: ____

Perineum Scar: Healthy/Not healthy

CLINICAL CHART OF BABY

Date: Temperature:																	
°F	**°C**																
104.0	40																
103.1	39.5																
102.2	39																
101.3	38.5																
100.4	38																
99.5	37.5																
98.6	37																
97.7	36.5																
96.8	36																
Heart Rate																	
Respiration																	
Urine																	
Stool																	
Vomit																	
Jaundice																	
Weight																	
Remarks																	

CLINICAL CHART OF PUERPERIUM

Date: Temperature:																	
°F	**°C**																
104.0	40																
103.1	39.5																
102.2	39																
101.3	38.5																
100.4	38																
99.5	37.5																
98.6	37																
97.7	36.5																
96.8	36																
95.9	35.5																
Respiration																	
BP																	
Lochia																	
Urine																	
Motion																	
Fundus in cm																	

Sign of Supervisor **Sign of Student**

POSTNATAL CARE

Name:__________ Age:______ G, P, L, A __________
Name of the Hospital:__________ Hospital Number: __________
Date of Delivery:__________ Date of Discharge:__________
Date of Registration:__________ LMP: ______ EDD: __________
Prenatal Record:__________ Gestation at 1st visit: __________

MEDICAL HISTORY

Chronic Illness:__________
Surgery:__________
Allergy:__________
Communicable Disease:__________

FAMILY HISTORY

Type of Family:
Nuclear:__________ Number of Persons:__________
Joint:__________ Number of Persons:__________

HISTORY OF MULTIPLE BIRTHS

Number of Children:__________ Girl Child:__________ Boy Child__________

SOCIOECONOMIC BACKGROUND

Religion:__________ Family Income:__________
Education: Husband:__________ Wife: __________
Occupation: Husband: __________ Wife: __________

DISEASES: Chronic Illness: ______ Genetic Disorder: ______ Psychiatric Disorder:______

MENSTRUAL HISTORY

Menarchy:______ Duration:______ Interval:______ Flow:______

MARITAL HISTORY

Age of marriage:__________ Year of Marriage: __________
Consanguineous: Yes/No

DIETARY PATTERN

Vegetarian:__________ Nonvegetarian: __________
Likes: __________ Dislikes: __________
Habits: Smoking/Drinking Alchohol/Chewing pan/Tobacco

PAST OBSTETRICAL HISTORY

S.No	Year	Full Term	Abortion	Type of Delivery	Sex of Baby	Alive	Stillbirth	Weight	Remarks

PRESENT PREGNANCY

Admission Notes:

Admission on:____________ at: ____________ Contractions Commenced:____________ at:____________________

Period of Gestation:____________________ Membranes: Intact:________________ Ruptured on:________________

Involution of Uterus:________________________________ Contractions________________________________

Presentation:____________________________________ Position:____________________________________

Engaged/Nonengaged:______________________________ FHR: ____________________________________

Bladder:____ Bowel: __________________________________

BP:____ TPR: ____________________________________

Special Observations:____

PRENATAL VISITS

Date of Booking	Weight	Height	Urine		BP	FHR	Weeks of Gestation	Height of Fundus	Position	Treatment
			Protein	Glucose						

GENERAL CONDITION

BP:________ TPR:__________________________ Urine: Sp. gavity__________________ Reaction:______________
Protein:_______________________ Glucose:____________________ Acetone:____________________________________

EXAMINATION AND INVESTIGATIONS

Blood Group:________ Rh Factor:_________ Hb:__________ VDRL:__________ HIV:__________Others:_______________
Heart_________ Lungs____________ Breast_____________ Abdomen________________ Perineum__________________

DELIVERY RECORD

Onset of True Labour: Date:_______________ Time:__________________
Time of Full Dilatation: Date:______________________ Time:_______________________
Membranes Ruptured at:_____________________ Spontaneous/Artificial: ______________ PROM:__________________

a. Delivery of Baby

Baby Born at:_________________ AM/PM, Male/Female:_____________ Mode of Delivery:______________________
Condition of Baby: Active/Nonactive/Asphyxiated _______________ Apgar Score _______________________________
Treatment: ____

b. Delivery of Placenta and Membranes

Delivery at:________________ AM/PM
Spontaneously/Manually removed____
Type of placenta____
Placenta and membranes: Complete/Incomplete____
Weight _____________ Cord Length___________________ Any Abnormality_______________________________
Total Blood Loss:____

c. Perineum

Intact___________ Episiotomy________________ Laceration_________________________ Repair_________________
Medications Given ____
____
____

d. Length of Labour

Mode of Delivery: ____

DURATION OF LABOUR

Progress of Labour	Date	Time	Total...... Hrs..... Min.....
Contraction Started			...... Hrs..... Min.....
Full Dilatation			
Delivery of Baby			...... Hrs..... Min.....
Delivery of Placenta			...... Hrs..... Min.....
Total Time Taken for Labour			

e. Condition of the Mother following Delivery

Pulse: ____________________ BP: ____________________ Uterus: Hard/Soft Vaginal bleeding: ____________________
Breastfeeding initiated at: ____
Perineum Scar: Healthy/Not healthy

CLINICAL CHART OF BABY

Date: Temperature:																	
°F	°C																
104.0	40																
103.1	39.5																
102.2	39																
101.3	38.5																
100.4	38																
99.5	37.5																
98.6	37																
97.7	36.5																
96.8	36																
Heart Rate																	
Respiration																	
Urine																	
Stool																	
Vomit																	
Jaundice																	
Weight																	
Remarks																	

CLINICAL CHART OF PUERPERIUM

Date: Temperature:																	
°F	**°C**																
104.0	40																
103.1	39.5																
102.2	39																
101.3	38.5																
100.4	38																
99.5	37.5																
98.6	37																
97.7	36.5																
96.8	36																
95.9	35.5																
Respiration																	
BP																	
Lochia																	
Urine																	
Motion																	
Fundus in cm																	

Sign of Supervisor **Sign of Student**

POSTNATAL CARE

Name:__________ Age:______ G, P, L, A __________
Name of the Hospital:__________ Hospital Number: __________
Date of Delivery:__________ Date of Discharge:__________
Date of Registration:__________ LMP: ______ EDD: __________
Prenatal Record:__________ Gestation at 1st visit: __________

MEDICAL HISTORY

Chronic Illness:__________
Surgery:__________
Allergy:__________
Communicable Disease:__________

FAMILY HISTORY

Type of Family:
Nuclear:__________ Number of Persons:__________
Joint:__________ Number of Persons:__________

HISTORY OF MULTIPLE BIRTHS

Number of Children:__________ Girl Child:________ Boy Child__________

SOCIOECONOMIC BACKGROUND

Religion:__________ Family Income:__________
Education: Husband:__________ Wife: __________
Occupation: Husband: __________ Wife: __________

DISEASES: Chronic Illness: ________ Genetic Disorder: ________ Psychiatric Disorder:________

MENSTRUAL HISTORY

Menarchy:__________ Duration:________ Interval:________ Flow:________

MARITAL HISTORY

Age of marriage:__________ Year of Marriage: __________
Consanguineous: Yes/No

DIETARY PATTERN

Vegetarian:__________ Nonvegetarian: __________
Likes: __________ Dislikes: __________
Habits: Smoking/Drinking Alchohol/Chewing pan/Tobacco

PAST OBSTETRICAL HISTORY

S.No	Year	Full Term	Abortion	Type of Delivery	Sex of Baby	Alive	Stillbirth	Weight	Remarks

PRESENT PREGNANCY

Admission Notes:

Admission on:____________ at:____________ Contractions Commenced:____________ at:____________

Period of Gestation:____________ Membranes: Intact:____________ Ruptured on:____________

Involution of Uterus:____________ Contractions____________

Presentation:____________ Position:____________

Engaged/Nonengaged:____________ FHR: ____________

Bladder:____________ Bowel: ____________

BP:____________ TPR: ____________

Special Observations:____________

PRENATAL VISITS

Date of Booking	Weight	Height	Urine		BP	FHR	Weeks of Gestation	Height of Fundus	Position	Treatment
			Protein	Glucose						

GENERAL CONDITION

BP:_________ TPR:__________________________ Urine: Sp. gavity__________________ Reaction:______________
Protein:_______________________ Glucose:____________________ Acetone:______________________________________

EXAMINATION AND INVESTIGATIONS

Blood Group:________ Rh Factor:_________ Hb:__________ VDRL:__________ HIV:__________Others:_______________
Heart_________ Lungs____________ Breast_____________ Abdomen________________ Perineum__________________

DELIVERY RECORD

Onset of True Labour: Date:_______________ Time:___________________
Time of Full Dilatation: Date:______________________ Time:________________________
Membranes Ruptured at:______________________ Spontaneous/Artificial: _______________ PROM:____________________

a. Delivery of Baby

Baby Born at:__________________ AM/PM, Male/Female:______________ Mode of Delivery:________________________
Condition of Baby: Active/Nonactive/Asphyxiated ________________ Apgar Score __________________________________
Treatment: ____

b. Delivery of Placenta and Membranes

Delivery at:__________________ AM/PM
Spontaneously/Manually removed____
Type of placenta____
Placenta and membranes: Complete/Incomplete____
Weight ______________ Cord Length____________________ Any Abnormality______________________________________
Total Blood Loss:____

c. Perineum

Intact___________ Episiotomy________________ Laceration_________________________ Repair__________________
Medications Given ____

d. Length of Labour

Mode of Delivery: ____

DURATION OF LABOUR

Progress of Labour	Date	Time	Total...... Hrs..... Min.....
Contraction Started			...... Hrs..... Min.....
Full Dilatation			
Delivery of Baby			...... Hrs..... Min.....
Delivery of Placenta			...... Hrs..... Min.....
Total Time Taken for Labour			

e. Condition of the Mother following Delivery

Pulse: ____________________BP:____________________ Uterus: Hard/Soft Vaginal bleeding: ____________________

Breastfeeding initiated at: ____

Perineum Scar: Healthy/Not healthy

CLINICAL CHART OF BABY

Date: Temperature:																	
°F	°C																
104.0	40																
103.1	39.5																
102.2	39																
101.3	38.5																
100.4	38																
99.5	37.5																
98.6	37																
97.7	36.5																
96.8	36																
Heart Rate																	
Respiration																	
Urine																	
Stool																	
Vomit																	
Jaundice																	
Weight																	
Remarks																	

CLINICAL CHART OF PUERPERIUM

Date: Temperature:																	
°F	°C																
104.0	40																
103.1	39.5																
102.2	39																
101.3	38.5																
100.4	38																
99.5	37.5																
98.6	37																
97.7	36.5																
96.8	36																
95.9	35.5																
Respiration																	
BP																	
Lochia																	
Urine																	
Motion																	
Fundus in cm																	

Sign of Supervisor **Sign of Student**

POSTNATAL CARE

Name:________________ Age:________ G, P, L, A ________________
Name of the Hospital:________________ Hospital Number: ________________
Date of Delivery:________________ Date of Discharge:________________
Date of Registration:________________ LMP: ________ EDD: ________________
Prenatal Record:________________ Gestation at 1st visit: ________________

MEDICAL HISTORY

Chronic Illness:________________
Surgery:________________
Allergy:________________
Communicable Disease:________________

FAMILY HISTORY

Type of Family:
Nuclear:________________ Number of Persons:________________
Joint:________________ Number of Persons:________________

HISTORY OF MULTIPLE BIRTHS

Number of Children:________________ Girl Child:________________ Boy Child________________

SOCIOECONOMIC BACKGROUND

Religion:________________ Family Income:________________
Education: Husband:________________ Wife: ________________
Occupation: Husband: ________________ Wife: ________________

DISEASES: Chronic Illness: ________ Genetic Disorder: ________ Psychiatric Disorder:________

MENSTRUAL HISTORY

Menarchy:________________Duration:________________Interval:________________Flow:________

MARITAL HISTORY

Age of marriage:________________ Year of Marriage: ________________
Consanguineous: Yes/No

DIETARY PATTERN

Vegetarian:________________ Nonvegetarian: ________________
Likes: ________________ Dislikes: ________________
Habits: Smoking/Drinking Alchohol/Chewing pan/Tobacco

PAST OBSTETRICAL HISTORY

S.No	Year	Full Term	Abortion	Type of Delivery	Sex of Baby	Alive	Stillbirth	Weight	Remarks

PRESENT PREGNANCY

Admission Notes:

Admission on:____________ at: ______________ Contractions Commenced:_____________ at:________________________

Period of Gestation:______________________ Membranes: Intact:__________________ Ruptured on:____________________

Involution of Uterus:________________________________ Contractions______________________________________

Presentation:_______________________________________ Position:____

Engaged/Nonengaged:_____________________________ FHR: ____

Bladder:____ Bowel: ____

BP:____ TPR: ____

Special Observations:____

PRENATAL VISITS

Date of Booking	Weight	Height	Urine		BP	FHR	Weeks of Gestation	Height of Fundus	Position	Treatment
			Protein	Glucose						

GENERAL CONDITION

BP:________ TPR:________________________ Urine: Sp. gavity________________ Reaction:____________

Protein:______________________ Glucose:__________________ Acetone:______________________________

EXAMINATION AND INVESTIGATIONS

Blood Group:_______ Rh Factor:________ Hb:_________ VDRL:_________ HIV:_________Others:______________

Heart_________ Lungs___________ Breast_____________ Abdomen_______________ Perineum________________

DELIVERY RECORD

Onset of True Labour: Date:______________ Time:_________________

Time of Full Dilatation: Date:_____________________ Time:______________________

Membranes Ruptured at:____________________ Spontaneous/Artificial: ______________ PROM:________________

a. Delivery of Baby

Baby Born at:_________________ AM/PM, Male/Female:_____________ Mode of Delivery:____________________

Condition of Baby: Active/Nonactive/Asphyxiated _______________ Apgar Score ________________________

Treatment: ____

b. Delivery of Placenta and Membranes

Delivery at:_______________ AM/PM

Spontaneously/Manually removed____

Type of placenta____

Placenta and membranes: Complete/Incomplete____

Weight ____________ Cord Length__________________ Any Abnormality_________________________

Total Blood Loss:____

c. Perineum

Intact__________ Episiotomy_______________ Laceration________________________ Repair________________

Medications Given ____

____

____

d. Length of Labour

Mode of Delivery: ____

DURATION OF LABOUR

Progress of Labour	Date	Time	Total...... Hrs..... Min.....
Contraction Started			...... Hrs..... Min.....
Full Dilatation			
Delivery of Baby			...... Hrs..... Min.....
Delivery of Placenta			...... Hrs..... Min.....
Total Time Taken for Labour			

e. Condition of the Mother following Delivery

Pulse: ___________________BP:___________________ Uterus: Hard/Soft Vaginal bleeding: ___________________

Breastfeeding initiated at: ____

Perineum Scar: Healthy/Not healthy

CLINICAL CHART OF BABY

Date: Temperature:																	
°F	°C																
104.0	40																
103.1	39.5																
102.2	39																
101.3	38.5																
100.4	38																
99.5	37.5																
98.6	37																
97.7	36.5																
96.8	36																
Heart Rate																	
Respiration																	
Urine																	
Stool																	
Vomit																	
Jaundice																	
Weight																	
Remarks																	

CLINICAL CHART OF PUERPERIUM

Date: Temperature:																	
°F	°C																
104.0	40																
103.1	39.5																
102.2	39																
101.3	38.5																
100.4	38																
99.5	37.5																
98.6	37																
97.7	36.5																
96.8	36																
95.9	35.5																
Respiration																	
BP																	
Lochia																	
Urine																	
Motion																	
Fundus in cm																	

Sign of Supervisor **Sign of Student**

POSTNATAL CARE

Name:__________ Age:__________ G, P, L, A __________
Name of the Hospital:__________ Hospital Number: __________
Date of Delivery:__________ Date of Discharge:__________
Date of Registration:__________ LMP: __________ EDD: __________
Prenatal Record:__________ Gestation at 1st visit: __________

MEDICAL HISTORY

Chronic Illness:__________
Surgery:__________
Allergy:__________
Communicable Disease:__________

FAMILY HISTORY

Type of Family:
Nuclear:__________ Number of Persons:__________
Joint:__________ Number of Persons:__________

HISTORY OF MULTIPLE BIRTHS

Number of Children:__________ Girl Child:__________ Boy Child__________

SOCIOECONOMIC BACKGROUND

Religion:__________ Family Income:__________
Education: Husband:__________ Wife: __________
Occupation: Husband: __________ Wife: __________

DISEASES: Chronic Illness: __________ Genetic Disorder: __________ Psychiatric Disorder:__________

MENSTRUAL HISTORY

Menarchy:__________ Duration:__________ Interval:__________ Flow:__________

MARITAL HISTORY

Age of marriage:__________ Year of Marriage: __________
Consanguineous: Yes/No

DIETARY PATTERN

Vegetarian:__________ Nonvegetarian: __________
Likes: __________ Dislikes: __________
Habits: Smoking/Drinking Alchohol/Chewing pan/Tobacco

PAST OBSTETRICAL HISTORY

S.No	Year	Full Term	Abortion	Type of Delivery	Sex of Baby	Alive	Stillbirth	Weight	Remarks

PRESENT PREGNANCY

Admission Notes:

Admission on:____________ at:_____________ Contractions Commenced:_____________ at:______________________
Period of Gestation:______________________ Membranes: Intact:_________________ Ruptured on:___________________
Involution of Uterus:_________________________________ Contractions____
Presentation:___________________________________ Position:____
Engaged/Nonengaged:________________________________ FHR: ____
Bladder:____ Bowel: ____
BP:____ TPR: ____

Special Observations:____

PRENATAL VISITS

Date of Booking	Weight	Height	Urine		BP	FHR	Weeks of Gestation	Height of Fundus	Position	Treatment
			Protein	Glucose						

GENERAL CONDITION

BP:_________ TPR:___________________________ Urine: Sp. gavity__________________ Reaction:______________
Protein:________________________ Glucose:____________________ Acetone:______________________________

EXAMINATION AND INVESTIGATIONS

Blood Group:________ Rh Factor:_________ Hb:__________ VDRL:__________ HIV:__________Others:_______________
Heart_________ Lungs_____________ Breast______________ Abdomen________________ Perineum___________________

DELIVERY RECORD

Onset of True Labour: Date:_______________ Time:__________________
Time of Full Dilatation: Date:______________________ Time:_________________________
Membranes Ruptured at:______________________ Spontaneous/Artificial: _______________ PROM:__________________

a. Delivery of Baby

Baby Born at:_________________ AM/PM, Male/Female:______________ Mode of Delivery:___________________
Condition of Baby: Active/Nonactive/Asphyxiated _______________ Apgar Score ___________________________
Treatment: ____

b. Delivery of Placenta and Membranes

Delivery at:________________ AM/PM
Spontaneously/Manually removed____
Type of placenta____
Placenta and membranes: Complete/Incomplete____
Weight _____________ Cord Length___________________ Any Abnormality_________________________
Total Blood Loss:____

c. Perineum

Intact___________ Episiotomy________________ Laceration_________________________ Repair__________________
Medications Given ____
____
____

d. Length of Labour

Mode of Delivery: ____

DURATION OF LABOUR

Progress of Labour	Date	Time	Total...... Hrs..... Min.....
Contraction Started			...... Hrs..... Min.....
Full Dilatation			
Delivery of Baby			...... Hrs..... Min.....
Delivery of Placenta			...... Hrs..... Min.....
Total Time Taken for Labour			

e. Condition of the Mother following Delivery

Pulse: __________________ BP: __________________ Uterus: Hard/Soft Vaginal bleeding: __________________
Breastfeeding initiated at: ____
Perineum Scar: Healthy/Not healthy

CLINICAL CHART OF BABY

Date: Temperature:																	
°F	°C																
104.0	40																
103.1	39.5																
102.2	39																
101.3	38.5																
100.4	38																
99.5	37.5																
98.6	37																
97.7	36.5																
96.8	36																
Heart Rate																	
Respiration																	
Urine																	
Stool																	
Vomit																	
Jaundice																	
Weight																	
Remarks																	

CLINICAL CHART OF PUERPERIUM

Date: Temperature:																	
°F	°C																
104.0	40																
103.1	39.5																
102.2	39																
101.3	38.5																
100.4	38																
99.5	37.5																
98.6	37																
97.7	36.5																
96.8	36																
95.9	35.5																
Respiration																	
BP																	
Lochia																	
Urine																	
Motion																	
Fundus in cm																	

Sign of Supervisor **Sign of Student**

POSTNATAL CARE

Name:__________ Age:__________ G, P, L, A __________
Name of the Hospital:__________ Hospital Number: __________
Date of Delivery:__________ Date of Discharge:__________
Date of Registration:__________ LMP: __________ EDD: __________
Prenatal Record:__________ Gestation at 1st visit: __________

MEDICAL HISTORY

Chronic Illness:__________
Surgery:__________
Allergy:__________
Communicable Disease:__________

FAMILY HISTORY

Type of Family:
Nuclear:__________ Number of Persons:__________
Joint:__________ Number of Persons:__________

HISTORY OF MULTIPLE BIRTHS

Number of Children:__________ Girl Child:__________ Boy Child__________

SOCIOECONOMIC BACKGROUND

Religion:__________ Family Income:__________
Education: Husband:__________ Wife: __________
Occupation: Husband: __________ Wife: __________

DISEASES: Chronic Illness: __________ Genetic Disorder: __________ Psychiatric Disorder:__________

MENSTRUAL HISTORY

Menarchy:__________Duration:__________Interval:__________Flow:__________

MARITAL HISTORY

Age of marriage:__________ Year of Marriage: __________
Consanguineous: Yes/No

DIETARY PATTERN

Vegetarian:__________ Nonvegetarian: __________
Likes: __________ Dislikes: __________
Habits: Smoking/Drinking Alchohol/Chewing pan/Tobacco

PAST OBSTETRICAL HISTORY

S.No	Year	Full Term	Abortion	Type of Delivery	Sex of Baby	Alive	Stillbirth	Weight	Remarks

PRESENT PREGNANCY

Admission Notes:

Admission on:____________ at: _____________ Contractions Commenced:_____________ at:____________________

Period of Gestation:______________________ Membranes: Intact:__________________ Ruptured on:__________________

Involution of Uterus:________________________________ Contractions____________________________________

Presentation:_______________________________________ Position:____

Engaged/Nonengaged:________________________________ FHR: ____

Bladder:____ Bowel: ____

BP:____ TPR: ____

Special Observations:____

PRENATAL VISITS

Date of Booking	Weight	Height	Urine		BP	FHR	Weeks of Gestation	Height of Fundus	Position	Treatment
			Protein	Glucose						

GENERAL CONDITION

BP:________ TPR:__________________________ Urine: Sp. gavity__________________ Reaction:______________
Protein:________________________Glucose:____________________Acetone:______________________________________

EXAMINATION AND INVESTIGATIONS

Blood Group:________ Rh Factor:_________ Hb:__________ VDRL:__________ HIV:__________Others:_______________
Heart_________ Lungs____________ Breast_____________ Abdomen________________ Perineum___________________

DELIVERY RECORD

Onset of True Labour: Date:_______________ Time:__________________
Time of Full Dilatation: Date:______________________ Time:________________________
Membranes Ruptured at:_____________________ Spontaneous/Artificial: ______________ PROM:_________________

a. Delivery of Baby

Baby Born at:_________________ AM/PM, Male/Female:_____________ Mode of Delivery:______________________
Condition of Baby: Active/Nonactive/Asphyxiated _______________ Apgar Score _____________________________
Treatment: ____

b. Delivery of Placenta and Membranes

Delivery at:________________ AM/PM
Spontaneously/Manually removed____
Type of placenta____
Placenta and membranes: Complete/Incomplete____
Weight _____________ Cord Length___________________ Any Abnormality_____________________________________
Total Blood Loss:____

c. Perineum

Intact___________ Episiotomy________________ Laceration_________________________ Repair__________________
Medications Given ____
____
____

d. Length of Labour

Mode of Delivery: ____

DURATION OF LABOUR

Progress of Labour	Date	Time	Total...... Hrs..... Min.....
Contraction Started			...... Hrs..... Min.....
Full Dilatation			
Delivery of Baby			...... Hrs..... Min.....
Delivery of Placenta			...... Hrs..... Min.....
Total Time Taken for Labour			

e. Condition of the Mother following Delivery

Pulse: ____________________ BP: ____________________ Uterus: Hard/Soft Vaginal bleeding: ____________________

Breastfeeding initiated at: ____

Perineum Scar: Healthy/Not healthy

CLINICAL CHART OF BABY

Date: Temperature:																	
°F	°C																
104.0	40																
103.1	39.5																
102.2	39																
101.3	38.5																
100.4	38																
99.5	37.5																
98.6	37																
97.7	36.5																
96.8	36																
Heart Rate																	
Respiration																	
Urine																	
Stool																	
Vomit																	
Jaundice																	
Weight																	
Remarks																	

CLINICAL CHART OF PUERPERIUM

Date: Temperature:																	
°F	**°C**																
104.0	40																
103.1	39.5																
102.2	39																
101.3	38.5																
100.4	38																
99.5	37.5																
98.6	37																
97.7	36.5																
96.8	36																
95.9	35.5																
Respiration																	
BP																	
Lochia																	
Urine																	
Motion																	
Fundus in cm																	

Sign of Supervisor **Sign of Student**

POSTNATAL CARE

Name:__________ Age:______ G, P, L, A __________
Name of the Hospital:__________ Hospital Number: __________
Date of Delivery:__________ Date of Discharge:__________
Date of Registration:__________ LMP: ______ EDD: __________
Prenatal Record:__________ Gestation at 1st visit: __________

MEDICAL HISTORY

Chronic Illness:__________
Surgery:__________
Allergy:__________
Communicable Disease:__________

FAMILY HISTORY

Type of Family:
Nuclear:__________ Number of Persons:__________
Joint:__________ Number of Persons:__________

HISTORY OF MULTIPLE BIRTHS

Number of Children:__________ Girl Child:______ Boy Child__________

SOCIOECONOMIC BACKGROUND

Religion:__________ Family Income:__________
Education: Husband:__________ Wife: __________
Occupation: Husband: __________ Wife: __________

DISEASES: Chronic Illness: ______ Genetic Disorder: ______ Psychiatric Disorder:______

MENSTRUAL HISTORY

Menarchy:______Duration:______Interval:______Flow:______

MARITAL HISTORY

Age of marriage:__________ Year of Marriage: __________
Consanguineous: Yes/No

DIETARY PATTERN

Vegetarian:__________ Nonvegetarian: __________
Likes: __________ Dislikes: __________
Habits: Smoking/Drinking Alchohol/Chewing pan/Tobacco

PAST OBSTETRICAL HISTORY

S.No	Year	Full Term	Abortion	Type of Delivery	Sex of Baby	Alive	Stillbirth	Weight	Remarks

PRESENT PREGNANCY

Admission Notes:

Admission on:__________ at:__________ Contractions Commenced:__________ at:__________
Period of Gestation:__________ Membranes: Intact:__________ Ruptured on:__________
Involution of Uterus:__________ Contractions__________
Presentation:__________ Position:__________
Engaged/Nonengaged:__________ FHR:__________
Bladder:__________ Bowel:__________
BP:__________ TPR:__________

Special Observations:__________

PRENATAL VISITS

Date of Booking	Weight	Height	Urine		BP	FHR	Weeks of Gestation	Height of Fundus	Position	Treatment
			Protein	Glucose						

GENERAL CONDITION

BP:__________ TPR:______________________________ Urine: Sp. gavity____________________ Reaction:________________
Protein:__________________________ Glucose:______________________ Acetone:____

EXAMINATION AND INVESTIGATIONS

Blood Group:_________ Rh Factor:__________ Hb:___________ VDRL:___________ HIV:___________Others:_________________
Heart__________ Lungs_____________ Breast_______________ Abdomen__________________ Perineum_____________________

DELIVERY RECORD

Onset of True Labour: Date:_________________ Time:___________________
Time of Full Dilatation: Date:_________________________ Time:__________________________
Membranes Ruptured at:________________________ Spontaneous/Artificial: ________________ PROM:______________________

a. Delivery of Baby

Baby Born at:____________________ AM/PM, Male/Female:_______________ Mode of Delivery:__________________________
Condition of Baby: Active/Nonactive/Asphyxiated _________________ Apgar Score ____________________________________
Treatment: ____

b. Delivery of Placenta and Membranes

Delivery at:__________________ AM/PM
Spontaneously/Manually removed____
Type of placenta____
Placenta and membranes: Complete/Incomplete____
Weight _______________ Cord Length_____________________ Any Abnormality____
Total Blood Loss:____

c. Perineum

Intact____________ Episiotomy_________________ Laceration___________________________ Repair____________________
Medications Given ____
____
____

d. Length of Labour

Mode of Delivery: ____

DURATION OF LABOUR

Progress of Labour	Date	Time	Total...... Hrs..... Min.....
Contraction Started			...... Hrs..... Min.....
Full Dilatation			
Delivery of Baby			...... Hrs..... Min.....
Delivery of Placenta			...... Hrs..... Min.....
Total Time Taken for Labour			

e. Condition of the Mother following Delivery

Pulse: ___________________BP:___________________ Uterus: Hard/Soft Vaginal bleeding: ___________________

Breastfeeding initiated at: ____

Perineum Scar: Healthy/Not healthy

CLINICAL CHART OF BABY

Date: Temperature:																	
°F	°C																
104.0	40																
103.1	39.5																
102.2	39																
101.3	38.5																
100.4	38																
99.5	37.5																
98.6	37																
97.7	36.5																
96.8	36																
Heart Rate																	
Respiration																	
Urine																	
Stool																	
Vomit																	
Jaundice																	
Weight																	
Remarks																	

CLINICAL CHART OF PUERPERIUM

Date: Temperature:																	
°F	°C																
104.0	40																
103.1	39.5																
102.2	39																
101.3	38.5																
100.4	38																
99.5	37.5																
98.6	37																
97.7	36.5																
96.8	36																
95.9	35.5																
Respiration																	
BP																	
Lochia																	
Urine																	
Motion																	
Fundus in cm																	

Sign of Supervisor **Sign of Student**

POSTNATAL CARE

Name:____________ Age:______ G, P, L, A ____________
Name of the Hospital:____________ Hospital Number: ____________
Date of Delivery:____________ Date of Discharge:____________
Date of Registration:____________ LMP: ______ EDD: ____________
Prenatal Record:____________ Gestation at 1st visit: ____________

MEDICAL HISTORY

Chronic Illness:____________
Surgery:____________
Allergy:____________
Communicable Disease:____________

FAMILY HISTORY

Type of Family:
Nuclear:____________ Number of Persons:____________
Joint:____________ Number of Persons:____________

HISTORY OF MULTIPLE BIRTHS

Number of Children:____________ Girl Child:________ Boy Child____________

SOCIOECONOMIC BACKGROUND

Religion:____________ Family Income:____________
Education: Husband:____________ Wife: ____________
Occupation: Husband: ____________ Wife: ____________

DISEASES: Chronic Illness: ________ Genetic Disorder: ________ Psychiatric Disorder:________

MENSTRUAL HISTORY

Menarchy:________ Duration:________ Interval:________ Flow:________

MARITAL HISTORY

Age of marriage:____________ Year of Marriage: ____________
Consanguineous: Yes/No

DIETARY PATTERN

Vegetarian:____________ Nonvegetarian: ____________
Likes: ____________ Dislikes: ____________
Habits: Smoking/Drinking Alchohol/Chewing pan/Tobacco

PAST OBSTETRICAL HISTORY

S.No	Year	Full Term	Abortion	Type of Delivery	Sex of Baby	Alive	Stillbirth	Weight	Remarks

PRESENT PREGNANCY

Admission Notes:

Admission on:____________ at:____________ Contractions Commenced:____________ at:____________
Period of Gestation:____________ Membranes: Intact:____________ Ruptured on:____________
Involution of Uterus:____________ Contractions____________
Presentation:____________ Position:____________
Engaged/Nonengaged:____________ FHR: ____________
Bladder:____________ Bowel: ____________
BP:____________ TPR: ____________

Special Observations:____________

PRENATAL VISITS

Date of Booking	Weight	Height	Urine		BP	FHR	Weeks of Gestation	Height of Fundus	Position	Treatment
			Protein	Glucose						

GENERAL CONDITION

BP:________ TPR:____________________ Urine: Sp. gavity______________ Reaction:___________
Protein:__________________ Glucose:_______________ Acetone:__________________________

EXAMINATION AND INVESTIGATIONS

Blood Group:_______ Rh Factor:_______ Hb:________ VDRL:________ HIV:________ Others:___________
Heart________ Lungs__________ Breast___________ Abdomen_____________ Perineum______________

DELIVERY RECORD

Onset of True Labour: Date:_____________ Time:______________
Time of Full Dilatation: Date:__________________ Time:__________________
Membranes Ruptured at:_________________ Spontaneous/Artificial: ___________ PROM:_______________

a. Delivery of Baby

Baby Born at:______________ AM/PM, Male/Female:___________ Mode of Delivery:_________________
Condition of Baby: Active/Nonactive/Asphyxiated ____________ Apgar Score _______________________
Treatment: ____

b. Delivery of Placenta and Membranes

Delivery at:_____________ AM/PM
Spontaneously/Manually removed____
Type of placenta____
Placenta and membranes: Complete/Incomplete____
Weight __________ Cord Length_______________ Any Abnormality_________________________
Total Blood Loss:____

c. Perineum

Intact_________ Episiotomy____________ Laceration____________________ Repair______________
Medications Given ____
____
____

d. Length of Labour

Mode of Delivery: ____

DURATION OF LABOUR

Progress of Labour	Date	Time	Total...... Hrs..... Min.....
Contraction Started			...... Hrs..... Min.....
Full Dilatation			
Delivery of Baby			...... Hrs..... Min.....
Delivery of Placenta			...... Hrs..... Min.....
Total Time Taken for Labour			

e. Condition of the Mother following Delivery

Pulse: ____________________BP:____________________ Uterus: Hard/Soft Vaginal bleeding: ____________________

Breastfeeding initiated at: ____

Perineum Scar: Healthy/Not healthy

CLINICAL CHART OF BABY

Date: Temperature:																	
°F	°C																
104.0	40																
103.1	39.5																
102.2	39																
101.3	38.5																
100.4	38																
99.5	37.5																
98.6	37																
97.7	36.5																
96.8	36																
Heart Rate																	
Respiration																	
Urine																	
Stool																	
Vomit																	
Jaundice																	
Weight																	
Remarks																	

CLINICAL CHART OF PUERPERIUM

Date: Temperature:																	
°F	°C																
104.0	40																
103.1	39.5																
102.2	39																
101.3	38.5																
100.4	38																
99.5	37.5																
98.6	37																
97.7	36.5																
96.8	36																
95.9	35.5																
Respiration																	
BP																	
Lochia																	
Urine																	
Motion																	
Fundus in cm																	

Sign of Supervisor **Sign of Student**

POSTNATAL CARE

Name:__________ Age:__________ G, P, L, A __________
Name of the Hospital:__________ Hospital Number: __________
Date of Delivery:__________ Date of Discharge:__________
Date of Registration:__________ LMP: __________ EDD: __________
Prenatal Record:__________ Gestation at 1st visit: __________

MEDICAL HISTORY

Chronic Illness:__________
Surgery:__________
Allergy:__________
Communicable Disease:__________

FAMILY HISTORY

Type of Family:
Nuclear:__________ Number of Persons:__________
Joint:__________ Number of Persons:__________

HISTORY OF MULTIPLE BIRTHS

Number of Children:__________ Girl Child:__________ Boy Child__________

SOCIOECONOMIC BACKGROUND

Religion:__________ Family Income:__________
Education: Husband:__________ Wife: __________
Occupation: Husband: __________ Wife: __________

DISEASES: Chronic Illness: __________ Genetic Disorder: __________ Psychiatric Disorder:__________

MENSTRUAL HISTORY

Menarchy:__________ Duration:__________ Interval:__________ Flow:__________

MARITAL HISTORY

Age of marriage:__________ Year of Marriage: __________
Consanguineous: Yes/No

DIETARY PATTERN

Vegetarian:__________ Nonvegetarian: __________
Likes: __________ Dislikes: __________
Habits: Smoking/Drinking Alchohol/Chewing pan/Tobacco

PAST OBSTETRICAL HISTORY

S.No	Year	Full Term	Abortion	Type of Delivery	Sex of Baby	Alive	Stillbirth	Weight	Remarks

PRESENT PREGNANCY

Admission Notes:

Admission on:____________ at:_____________ Contractions Commenced:_____________ at:______________________

Period of Gestation:_____________________ Membranes: Intact:_________________ Ruptured on:_____________________

Involution of Uterus:__________________________________ Contractions_____________________________________

Presentation:_______________________________________ Position:______________________________________

Engaged/Nonengaged:________________________________ FHR: _______________________________________

Bladder:____ Bowel: _________________________________

BP:____ TPR: ______________________________________

Special Observations:____

PRENATAL VISITS

Date of Booking	Weight	Height	Urine		BP	FHR	Weeks of Gestation	Height of Fundus	Position	Treatment
			Protein	Glucose						

GENERAL CONDITION

BP:________ TPR:________________________ Urine: Sp. gavity________________ Reaction:____________
Protein:______________________ Glucose:___________________ Acetone:____________________________________

EXAMINATION AND INVESTIGATIONS

Blood Group:________ Rh Factor:_________ Hb:__________ VDRL:__________ HIV:__________Others:_______________
Heart_________ Lungs____________ Breast_____________ Abdomen________________ Perineum__________________

DELIVERY RECORD

Onset of True Labour: Date:_______________ Time:__________________
Time of Full Dilatation: Date:_____________________ Time:______________________
Membranes Ruptured at:____________________ Spontaneous/Artificial: ______________ PROM:__________________

a. Delivery of Baby

Baby Born at:_________________ AM/PM, Male/Female:_____________ Mode of Delivery:______________________
Condition of Baby: Active/Nonactive/Asphyxiated _______________ Apgar Score ______________________________
Treatment: ____

b. Delivery of Placenta and Membranes

Delivery at:________________ AM/PM
Spontaneously/Manually removed____
Type of placenta____
Placenta and membranes: Complete/Incomplete____
Weight _____________ Cord Length__________________ Any Abnormality____________________________________
Total Blood Loss:____

c. Perineum

Intact___________ Episiotomy_______________ Laceration________________________ Repair_________________
Medications Given ____
____
____

d. Length of Labour

Mode of Delivery: ____

DURATION OF LABOUR

Progress of Labour	Date	Time	Total...... Hrs..... Min.....
Contraction Started			...... Hrs..... Min.....
Full Dilatation			
Delivery of Baby			...... Hrs..... Min.....
Delivery of Placenta			...... Hrs..... Min.....
Total Time Taken for Labour			

e. Condition of the Mother following Delivery

Pulse: ____________________ BP: ____________________ Uterus: Hard/Soft Vaginal bleeding: ____________________

Breastfeeding initiated at: ____

Perineum Scar: Healthy/Not healthy

CLINICAL CHART OF BABY

Date: Temperature:																	
°F	**°C**																
104.0	40																
103.1	39.5																
102.2	39																
101.3	38.5																
100.4	38																
99.5	37.5																
98.6	37																
97.7	36.5																
96.8	36																
Heart Rate																	
Respiration																	
Urine																	
Stool																	
Vomit																	
Jaundice																	
Weight																	
Remarks																	

CLINICAL CHART OF PUERPERIUM

Date: Temperature:																	
°F	**°C**																
104.0	40																
103.1	39.5																
102.2	39																
101.3	38.5																
100.4	38																
99.5	37.5																
98.6	37																
97.7	36.5																
96.8	36																
95.9	35.5																
Respiration																	
BP																	
Lochia																	
Urine																	
Motion																	
Fundus in cm																	

Sign of Supervisor **Sign of Student**

POSTNATAL CARE

Name:______________________ Age:__________ G, P, L, A ______________________
Name of the Hospital:______________________ Hospital Number: ______________________
Date of Delivery:______________________ Date of Discharge:______________________
Date of Registration:______________________ LMP: __________ EDD: ______________________
Prenatal Record:______________________ Gestation at 1st visit: ______________________

MEDICAL HISTORY

Chronic Illness:______________________
Surgery:______________________
Allergy:______________________
Communicable Disease:______________________

FAMILY HISTORY

Type of Family:
Nuclear:______________________ Number of Persons:______________________
Joint:______________________ Number of Persons:______________________

HISTORY OF MULTIPLE BIRTHS

Number of Children:______________________ Girl Child:______________ Boy Child______________________

SOCIOECONOMIC BACKGROUND

Religion:______________________ Family Income:______________________
Education: Husband:______________________ Wife: ______________________
Occupation: Husband: ______________________ Wife: ______________________

DISEASES: Chronic Illness: ______________ Genetic Disorder: ______________ Psychiatric Disorder:______________

MENSTRUAL HISTORY

Menarchy:______________ Duration:______________ Interval:______________ Flow:______________

MARITAL HISTORY

Age of marriage:______________________ Year of Marriage: ______________________
Consanguineous: Yes/No

DIETARY PATTERN

Vegetarian:______________________ Nonvegetarian: ______________________
Likes: ______________________ Dislikes: ______________________
Habits: Smoking/Drinking Alchohol/Chewing pan/Tobacco

PAST OBSTETRICAL HISTORY

S.No	Year	Full Term	Abortion	Type of Delivery	Sex of Baby	Alive	Stillbirth	Weight	Remarks

PRESENT PREGNANCY

Admission Notes:

Admission on:__________ at:__________ Contractions Commenced:__________ at:__________
Period of Gestation:__________ Membranes: Intact:__________ Ruptured on:__________
Involution of Uterus:__________ Contractions__________
Presentation:__________ Position:__________
Engaged/Nonengaged:__________ FHR:__________
Bladder:__________ Bowel:__________
BP:__________ TPR:__________

Special Observations:__________

PRENATAL VISITS

Date of Booking	Weight	Height	Urine		BP	FHR	Weeks of Gestation	Height of Fundus	Position	Treatment
			Protein	Glucose						

GENERAL CONDITION

BP:_________ TPR:___________________________ Urine: Sp. gavity___________________ Reaction:______________
Protein:________________________ Glucose:_____________________ Acetone:__________________________________

EXAMINATION AND INVESTIGATIONS

Blood Group:________ Rh Factor:_________ Hb:__________ VDRL:__________ HIV:__________Others:_______________
Heart_________ Lungs____________ Breast_____________ Abdomen_________________ Perineum___________________

DELIVERY RECORD

Onset of True Labour: Date:_______________ Time:___________________
Time of Full Dilatation: Date:______________________ Time:________________________
Membranes Ruptured at:______________________ Spontaneous/Artificial: _______________ PROM:___________________

a. Delivery of Baby

Baby Born at:__________________ AM/PM, Male/Female:______________ Mode of Delivery:_______________________
Condition of Baby: Active/Nonactive/Asphyxiated ________________ Apgar Score _________________________________
Treatment: ____

b. Delivery of Placenta and Membranes

Delivery at:_________________ AM/PM
Spontaneously/Manually removed____
Type of placenta____
Placenta and membranes: Complete/Incomplete____
Weight _____________ Cord Length____________________ Any Abnormality______________________________________
Total Blood Loss:____

c. Perineum

Intact___________ Episiotomy________________ Laceration__________________________ Repair__________________
Medications Given ____
____
____

d. Length of Labour

Mode of Delivery: ____

DURATION OF LABOUR

Progress of Labour	Date	Time	Total...... Hrs..... Min.....
Contraction Started			...... Hrs..... Min.....
Full Dilatation			
Delivery of Baby			...... Hrs..... Min.....
Delivery of Placenta			...... Hrs..... Min.....
Total Time Taken for Labour			

e. Condition of the Mother following Delivery

Pulse: ___________________BP:___________________ Uterus: Hard/Soft Vaginal bleeding: ___________________

Breastfeeding initiated at: ____

Perineum Scar: Healthy/Not healthy

CLINICAL CHART OF BABY

Date: Temperature:																	
°F	°C																
104.0	40																
103.1	39.5																
102.2	39																
101.3	38.5																
100.4	38																
99.5	37.5																
98.6	37																
97.7	36.5																
96.8	36																
Heart Rate																	
Respiration																	
Urine																	
Stool																	
Vomit																	
Jaundice																	
Weight																	
Remarks																	

CLINICAL CHART OF PUERPERIUM

Date: Temperature:																	
°F	**°C**																
104.0	40																
103.1	39.5																
102.2	39																
101.3	38.5																
100.4	38																
99.5	37.5																
98.6	37																
97.7	36.5																
96.8	36																
95.9	35.5																
Respiration																	
BP																	
Lochia																	
Urine																	
Motion																	
Fundus in cm																	

Sign of Supervisor **Sign of Student**

POSTNATAL CARE

Name:______________ Age:________ G, P, L, A ______________
Name of the Hospital:______________ Hospital Number: ______________
Date of Delivery:______________ Date of Discharge:______________
Date of Registration:______________ LMP: ________ EDD: ______________
Prenatal Record:______________ Gestation at 1st visit: ______________

MEDICAL HISTORY

Chronic Illness:______________
Surgery:______________
Allergy:______________
Communicable Disease:______________

FAMILY HISTORY

Type of Family:
Nuclear:______________ Number of Persons:______________
Joint:______________ Number of Persons:______________

HISTORY OF MULTIPLE BIRTHS

Number of Children:______________ Girl Child:__________ Boy Child______________

SOCIOECONOMIC BACKGROUND

Religion:______________ Family Income:______________
Education: Husband:______________ Wife: ______________
Occupation: Husband: ______________ Wife: ______________

DISEASES: Chronic Illness: __________ Genetic Disorder: __________ Psychiatric Disorder:______________

MENSTRUAL HISTORY

Menarchy:__________ Duration:__________ Interval:__________ Flow:__________

MARITAL HISTORY

Age of marriage:______________ Year of Marriage: ______________
Consanguineous: Yes/No

DIETARY PATTERN

Vegetarian:______________ Nonvegetarian: ______________
Likes: ______________ Dislikes: ______________
Habits: Smoking/Drinking Alchohol/Chewing pan/Tobacco

PAST OBSTETRICAL HISTORY

S.No	Year	Full Term	Abortion	Type of Delivery	Sex of Baby	Alive	Stillbirth	Weight	Remarks

PRESENT PREGNANCY

Admission Notes:

Admission on:__________ at:__________ Contractions Commenced:__________ at:__________

Period of Gestation:__________ Membranes: Intact:__________ Ruptured on:__________

Involution of Uterus:__________ Contractions__________

Presentation:__________ Position:__________

Engaged/Nonengaged:__________ FHR:__________

Bladder:__________ Bowel:__________

BP:__________ TPR:__________

Special Observations:__________

PRENATAL VISITS

Date of Booking	Weight	Height	Urine		BP	FHR	Weeks of Gestation	Height of Fundus	Position	Treatment
			Protein	Glucose						

GENERAL CONDITION

BP:________ TPR:__________________________ Urine: Sp. gavity_________________ Reaction:______________
Protein:_______________________Glucose:____________________ Acetone:___________________________________

EXAMINATION AND INVESTIGATIONS

Blood Group:________ Rh Factor:_________ Hb:__________ VDRL:__________ HIV:__________Others:________________
Heart_________ Lungs____________ Breast_____________ Abdomen________________ Perineum__________________

DELIVERY RECORD

Onset of True Labour: Date:_______________ Time:__________________
Time of Full Dilatation: Date:______________________ Time:________________________
Membranes Ruptured at:_____________________ Spontaneous/Artificial: ______________ PROM:__________________

a. Delivery of Baby

Baby Born at:_________________ AM/PM, Male/Female:_____________ Mode of Delivery:____________________
Condition of Baby: Active/Nonactive/Asphyxiated _______________ Apgar Score ____________________________
Treatment: ____

b. Delivery of Placenta and Membranes

Delivery at:________________ AM/PM
Spontaneously/Manually removed____
Type of placenta____
Placenta and membranes: Complete/Incomplete____
Weight _____________ Cord Length___________________ Any Abnormality__________________________
Total Blood Loss:____

c. Perineum

Intact___________ Episiotomy________________ Laceration_________________________ Repair__________________
Medications Given ____
____
____

d. Length of Labour

Mode of Delivery: ____

DURATION OF LABOUR

Progress of Labour	Date	Time	Total...... Hrs..... Min.....
Contraction Started			...... Hrs..... Min.....
Full Dilatation			
Delivery of Baby			...... Hrs..... Min.....
Delivery of Placenta			...... Hrs..... Min.....
Total Time Taken for Labour			

e. Condition of the Mother following Delivery

Pulse: __________________BP:__________________ Uterus: Hard/Soft Vaginal bleeding: __________________

Breastfeeding initiated at: ____

Perineum Scar: Healthy/Not healthy

CLINICAL CHART OF BABY

Date: Temperature:																	
°F	**°C**																
104.0	40																
103.1	39.5																
102.2	39																
101.3	38.5																
100.4	38																
99.5	37.5																
98.6	37																
97.7	36.5																
96.8	36																
Heart Rate																	
Respiration																	
Urine																	
Stool																	
Vomit																	
Jaundice																	
Weight																	
Remarks																	

CLINICAL CHART OF PUERPERIUM

Date: Temperature:																	
°F	°C																
104.0	40																
103.1	39.5																
102.2	39																
101.3	38.5																
100.4	38																
99.5	37.5																
98.6	37																
97.7	36.5																
96.8	36																
95.9	35.5																
Respiration																	
BP																	
Lochia																	
Urine																	
Motion																	
Fundus in cm																	

Sign of Supervisor **Sign of Student**

POSTNATAL CARE

Name:______________________ Age:__________ G, P, L, A ______________________
Name of the Hospital:______________________ Hospital Number: ______________________
Date of Delivery:______________________ Date of Discharge:______________________
Date of Registration:______________________ LMP: __________ EDD: ______________________
Prenatal Record:______________________ Gestation at 1st visit: ______________________

MEDICAL HISTORY

Chronic Illness:______________________
Surgery:______________________
Allergy:______________________
Communicable Disease:______________________

FAMILY HISTORY

Type of Family:
Nuclear:______________________ Number of Persons:______________________
Joint:______________________ Number of Persons:______________________

HISTORY OF MULTIPLE BIRTHS

Number of Children:______________________ Girl Child:______________ Boy Child______________________

SOCIOECONOMIC BACKGROUND

Religion:______________________ Family Income:______________________
Education: Husband:______________________ Wife: ______________________
Occupation: Husband: ______________________ Wife: ______________________

DISEASES: Chronic Illness: ____________ Genetic Disorder: ____________ Psychiatric Disorder:______________

MENSTRUAL HISTORY

Menarchy:______________Duration:______________Interval:______________Flow:__________

MARITAL HISTORY

Age of marriage:______________________ Year of Marriage: ______________________
Consanguineous: Yes/No

DIETARY PATTERN

Vegetarian:______________________ Nonvegetarian: ______________________
Likes: ______________________ Dislikes: ______________________
Habits: Smoking/Drinking Alchohol/Chewing pan/Tobacco

PAST OBSTETRICAL HISTORY

S.No	Year	Full Term	Abortion	Type of Delivery	Sex of Baby	Alive	Stillbirth	Weight	Remarks

PRESENT PREGNANCY

Admission Notes:

Admission on:____________ at:____________ Contractions Commenced:____________ at:____________

Period of Gestation:____________ Membranes: Intact:____________ Ruptured on:____________

Involution of Uterus:____________ Contractions____________

Presentation:____________ Position:____________

Engaged/Nonengaged:____________ FHR: ____________

Bladder:____________ Bowel: ____________

BP:____________ TPR: ____________

Special Observations:____________

PRENATAL VISITS

Date of Booking	Weight	Height	Urine		BP	FHR	Weeks of Gestation	Height of Fundus	Position	Treatment
			Protein	Glucose						

GENERAL CONDITION

BP:________ TPR:________________________ Urine: Sp. gavity________________ Reaction:____________
Protein:______________________ Glucose:___________________ Acetone:______________________________

EXAMINATION AND INVESTIGATIONS

Blood Group:________ Rh Factor:________ Hb:_________ VDRL:_________ HIV:_________Others:______________
Heart_________ Lungs____________ Breast_____________ Abdomen________________ Perineum__________________

DELIVERY RECORD

Onset of True Labour: Date:______________ Time:_________________
Time of Full Dilatation: Date:_____________________ Time:______________________
Membranes Ruptured at:____________________ Spontaneous/Artificial: ______________ PROM:____________________

a. Delivery of Baby

Baby Born at:________________ AM/PM, Male/Female:_____________ Mode of Delivery:______________________
Condition of Baby: Active/Nonactive/Asphyxiated _______________ Apgar Score _____________________________
Treatment: ____

b. Delivery of Placenta and Membranes

Delivery at:_______________ AM/PM
Spontaneously/Manually removed____
Type of placenta____
Placenta and membranes: Complete/Incomplete____
Weight _____________ Cord Length__________________ Any Abnormality_____________________________________
Total Blood Loss:____

c. Perineum

Intact___________ Episiotomy________________ Laceration________________________ Repair________________
Medications Given ____
____
____

d. Length of Labour

Mode of Delivery: ____

DURATION OF LABOUR

Progress of Labour	Date	Time	Total...... Hrs..... Min.....
Contraction Started			...... Hrs..... Min.....
Full Dilatation			
Delivery of Baby			...... Hrs..... Min.....
Delivery of Placenta			...... Hrs..... Min.....
Total Time Taken for Labour			

e. Condition of the Mother following Delivery

Pulse: ____________________BP:____________________ Uterus: Hard/Soft Vaginal bleeding: ____________________

Breastfeeding initiated at: ____

Perineum Scar: Healthy/Not healthy

CLINICAL CHART OF BABY

Date: Temperature:																	
°F	**°C**																
104.0	40																
103.1	39.5																
102.2	39																
101.3	38.5																
100.4	38																
99.5	37.5																
98.6	37																
97.7	36.5																
96.8	36																
Heart Rate																	
Respiration																	
Urine																	
Stool																	
Vomit																	
Jaundice																	
Weight																	
Remarks																	

CLINICAL CHART OF PUERPERIUM

Date: Temperature:																	
°F	**°C**																
104.0	40																
103.1	39.5																
102.2	39																
101.3	38.5																
100.4	38																
99.5	37.5																
98.6	37																
97.7	36.5																
96.8	36																
95.9	35.5																
Respiration																	
BP																	
Lochia																	
Urine																	
Motion																	
Fundus in cm																	

Sign of Supervisor **Sign of Student**

POSTNATAL CARE

Name:________________ Age:________ G, P, L, A ________________
Name of the Hospital:________________ Hospital Number: ________________
Date of Delivery:________________ Date of Discharge:________________
Date of Registration:________________ LMP: ________ EDD: ________________
Prenatal Record:________________ Gestation at 1st visit: ________________

MEDICAL HISTORY

Chronic Illness:________________
Surgery:________________
Allergy:________________
Communicable Disease:________________

FAMILY HISTORY

Type of Family:
Nuclear:________________ Number of Persons:________________
Joint:________________ Number of Persons:________________

HISTORY OF MULTIPLE BIRTHS

Number of Children:________________ Girl Child:________________ Boy Child________________

SOCIOECONOMIC BACKGROUND

Religion:________________ Family Income:________________
Education: Husband:________________ Wife: ________________
Occupation: Husband: ________________ Wife: ________________

DISEASES: Chronic Illness: ________ Genetic Disorder: ________ Psychiatric Disorder:________

MENSTRUAL HISTORY

Menarchy:________ Duration:________ Interval:________ Flow:________

MARITAL HISTORY

Age of marriage:________________ Year of Marriage: ________________
Consanguineous: Yes/No

DIETARY PATTERN

Vegetarian:________________ Nonvegetarian: ________________
Likes: ________________ Dislikes: ________________
Habits: Smoking/Drinking Alchohol/Chewing pan/Tobacco

PAST OBSTETRICAL HISTORY

S.No	Year	Full Term	Abortion	Type of Delivery	Sex of Baby	Alive	Stillbirth	Weight	Remarks

PRESENT PREGNANCY

Admission Notes:

Admission on:_____________ at:______________ Contractions Commenced:_____________ at:____________________

Period of Gestation:______________________ Membranes: Intact:__________________ Ruptured on:__________________

Involution of Uterus:________________________________ Contractions____________________________________

Presentation:_____________________________________ Position:_______________________________________

Engaged/Nonengaged:______________________________ FHR: _______________________________________

Bladder:____ Bowel: _______________________________________

BP:____ TPR: ____

Special Observations:____

PRENATAL VISITS

Date of Booking	Weight	Height	Urine		BP	FHR	Weeks of Gestation	Height of Fundus	Position	Treatment
			Protein	Glucose						

GENERAL CONDITION

BP:________ TPR:________________________ Urine: Sp. gavity________________ Reaction:____________
Protein:______________________ Glucose:__________________ Acetone:________________________________

EXAMINATION AND INVESTIGATIONS

Blood Group:________ Rh Factor:_________ Hb:__________ VDRL:__________ HIV:__________Others:______________
Heart_________ Lungs____________ Breast______________ Abdomen_______________ Perineum__________________

DELIVERY RECORD

Onset of True Labour: Date:______________ Time:__________________
Time of Full Dilatation: Date:____________________ Time:______________________
Membranes Ruptured at:____________________ Spontaneous/Artificial: ______________ PROM:__________________

a. Delivery of Baby

Baby Born at:________________ AM/PM, Male/Female:____________ Mode of Delivery:__________________
Condition of Baby: Active/Nonactive/Asphyxiated ______________ Apgar Score ____________________________
Treatment: ____

b. Delivery of Placenta and Membranes

Delivery at:_______________ AM/PM
Spontaneously/Manually removed____
Type of placenta____
Placenta and membranes: Complete/Incomplete____
Weight ____________ Cord Length_________________ Any Abnormality____________________________
Total Blood Loss:____

c. Perineum

Intact__________ Episiotomy______________ Laceration______________________ Repair_______________
Medications Given ____
____
____

d. Length of Labour

Mode of Delivery: ____

DURATION OF LABOUR

<table>
<tr><th>Progress of Labour</th><th>Date</th><th>Time</th><th>Total...... Hrs..... Min.....</th></tr>
<tr><td>Contraction Started</td><td></td><td></td><td rowspan="2">...... Hrs..... Min.....</td></tr>
<tr><td>Full Dilatation</td><td></td><td></td></tr>
<tr><td>Delivery of Baby</td><td></td><td></td><td>...... Hrs..... Min.....</td></tr>
<tr><td>Delivery of Placenta</td><td></td><td></td><td>...... Hrs..... Min.....</td></tr>
<tr><td>Total Time Taken for Labour</td><td></td><td></td><td></td></tr>
</table>

e. Condition of the Mother following Delivery

Pulse: ____________________BP:____________________ Uterus: Hard/Soft Vaginal bleeding: ____________________

Breastfeeding initiated at: ____

Perineum Scar: Healthy/Not healthy

CLINICAL CHART OF BABY

Date: Temperature:																	
°F	**°C**																
104.0	40																
103.1	39.5																
102.2	39																
101.3	38.5																
100.4	38																
99.5	37.5																
98.6	37																
97.7	36.5																
96.8	36																
Heart Rate																	
Respiration																	
Urine																	
Stool																	
Vomit																	
Jaundice																	
Weight																	
Remarks																	

CLINICAL CHART OF PUERPERIUM

Date: Temperature:																	
°F	°C																
104.0	40																
103.1	39.5																
102.2	39																
101.3	38.5																
100.4	38																
99.5	37.5																
98.6	37																
97.7	36.5																
96.8	36																
95.9	35.5																
Respiration																	
BP																	
Lochia																	
Urine																	
Motion																	
Fundus in cm																	

Sign of Supervisor **Sign of Student**

POSTNATAL CARE

Name:________________ Age:________ G, P, L, A ________________
Name of the Hospital:________________ Hospital Number: ________________
Date of Delivery:________________ Date of Discharge:________________
Date of Registration:________________ LMP: ________ EDD: ________________
Prenatal Record:________________ Gestation at 1st visit: ________________

MEDICAL HISTORY

Chronic Illness:________________
Surgery:________________
Allergy:________________
Communicable Disease:________________

FAMILY HISTORY

Type of Family:
Nuclear:________________ Number of Persons:________________
Joint:________________ Number of Persons:________________

HISTORY OF MULTIPLE BIRTHS

Number of Children:________________ Girl Child:____________ Boy Child________________

SOCIOECONOMIC BACKGROUND

Religion:________________ Family Income:________________
Education: Husband:________________ Wife: ________________
Occupation: Husband: ________________ Wife: ________________

DISEASES: Chronic Illness: __________ Genetic Disorder: __________ Psychiatric Disorder:__________

MENSTRUAL HISTORY

Menarchy:____________Duration:____________Interval:____________Flow:________

MARITAL HISTORY

Age of marriage:________________ Year of Marriage: ________________
Consanguineous: Yes/No

DIETARY PATTERN

Vegetarian:____________ Nonvegetarian: ________________
Likes: ________________ Dislikes: ________________
Habits: Smoking/Drinking Alchohol/Chewing pan/Tobacco

PAST OBSTETRICAL HISTORY

S.No	Year	Full Term	Abortion	Type of Delivery	Sex of Baby	Alive	Stillbirth	Weight	Remarks

PRESENT PREGNANCY

Admission Notes:

Admission on:__________ at: __________ Contractions Commenced:__________ at:__________
Period of Gestation:__________ Membranes: Intact:__________ Ruptured on:__________
Involution of Uterus:__________ Contractions__________
Presentation:__________ Position:__________
Engaged/Nonengaged:__________ FHR: __________
Bladder:__________ Bowel: __________
BP:__________ TPR: __________

Special Observations:__________

PRENATAL VISITS

Date of Booking	Weight	Height	Urine		BP	FHR	Weeks of Gestation	Height of Fundus	Position	Treatment
			Protein	Glucose						

GENERAL CONDITION

BP:_________ TPR:___________________________ Urine: Sp. gavity___________________ Reaction:______________
Protein:________________________ Glucose:_____________________ Acetone:________________________________

EXAMINATION AND INVESTIGATIONS

Blood Group:________ Rh Factor:_________ Hb:__________ VDRL:__________ HIV:__________Others:_______________
Heart_________ Lungs____________ Breast_____________ Abdomen________________ Perineum__________________

DELIVERY RECORD

Onset of True Labour: Date:________________ Time:___________________
Time of Full Dilatation: Date:______________________ Time:________________________
Membranes Ruptured at:______________________ Spontaneous/Artificial: _______________ PROM:___________________

a. Delivery of Baby

Baby Born at:__________________ AM/PM, Male/Female:_____________ Mode of Delivery:______________________
Condition of Baby: Active/Nonactive/Asphyxiated ________________ Apgar Score _____________________________
Treatment: ____

b. Delivery of Placenta and Membranes

Delivery at:________________ AM/PM
Spontaneously/Manually removed____
Type of placenta____
Placenta and membranes: Complete/Incomplete____
Weight ______________ Cord Length____________________ Any Abnormality______________________________
Total Blood Loss:____

c. Perineum

Intact___________ Episiotomy________________ Laceration_________________________ Repair___________________
Medications Given ____
____
____

d. Length of Labour

Mode of Delivery: ____

DURATION OF LABOUR

Progress of Labour	Date	Time	Total...... Hrs..... Min.....
Contraction Started			...... Hrs..... Min.....
Full Dilatation			
Delivery of Baby			...... Hrs..... Min.....
Delivery of Placenta			...... Hrs..... Min.....
Total Time Taken for Labour			

e. Condition of the Mother following Delivery

Pulse: ____________________BP:____________________ Uterus: Hard/Soft Vaginal bleeding: ____________________

Breastfeeding initiated at: ____

Perineum Scar: Healthy/Not healthy

CLINICAL CHART OF BABY

Date: Temperature:																	
°F	°C																
104.0	40																
103.1	39.5																
102.2	39																
101.3	38.5																
100.4	38																
99.5	37.5																
98.6	37																
97.7	36.5																
96.8	36																
Heart Rate																	
Respiration																	
Urine																	
Stool																	
Vomit																	
Jaundice																	
Weight																	
Remarks																	

CLINICAL CHART OF PUERPERIUM

Date: Temperature:																	
°F	**°C**																
104.0	40																
103.1	39.5																
102.2	39																
101.3	38.5																
100.4	38																
99.5	37.5																
98.6	37																
97.7	36.5																
96.8	36																
95.9	35.5																
Respiration																	
BP																	
Lochia																	
Urine																	
Motion																	
Fundus in cm																	

Sign of Supervisor **Sign of Student**

POSTNATAL CARE

Name:____________________ Age:__________ G, P, L, A ____________________
Name of the Hospital:____________________ Hospital Number: ____________________
Date of Delivery:____________________ Date of Discharge:____________________
Date of Registration:____________________ LMP: __________ EDD: ____________________
Prenatal Record:____________________ Gestation at 1st visit: ____________________

MEDICAL HISTORY

Chronic Illness:____________________
Surgery:____________________
Allergy:____________________
Communicable Disease:____________________

FAMILY HISTORY

Type of Family:
Nuclear:____________________ Number of Persons:____________________
Joint:____________________ Number of Persons:____________________

HISTORY OF MULTIPLE BIRTHS

Number of Children:____________________ Girl Child:__________ Boy Child____________________

SOCIOECONOMIC BACKGROUND

Religion:____________________ Family Income:____________________
Education: Husband:____________________ Wife: ____________________
Occupation: Husband: ____________________ Wife: ____________________

DISEASES: Chronic Illness: __________ Genetic Disorder: __________ Psychiatric Disorder:__________

MENSTRUAL HISTORY

Menarchy:__________ Duration:__________ Interval:__________ Flow:__________

MARITAL HISTORY

Age of marriage:____________________ Year of Marriage: ____________________
Consanguineous: Yes/No

DIETARY PATTERN

Vegetarian:____________________ Nonvegetarian: ____________________
Likes: ____________________ Dislikes: ____________________
Habits: Smoking/Drinking Alchohol/Chewing pan/Tobacco

PAST OBSTETRICAL HISTORY

S.No	Year	Full Term	Abortion	Type of Delivery	Sex of Baby	Alive	Stillbirth	Weight	Remarks

PRESENT PREGNANCY

Admission Notes:

Admission on:____________ at:____________ Contractions Commenced:____________ at:____________

Period of Gestation:____________ Membranes: Intact:____________ Ruptured on:____________

Involution of Uterus:____________ Contractions____________

Presentation:____________ Position:____________

Engaged/Nonengaged:____________ FHR: ____________

Bladder:____________ Bowel: ____________

BP:____________ TPR: ____________

Special Observations:____________

PRENATAL VISITS

Date of Booking	Weight	Height	Urine		BP	FHR	Weeks of Gestation	Height of Fundus	Position	Treatment
			Protein	Glucose						

GENERAL CONDITION

BP:________ TPR:__________________________ Urine: Sp. gavity__________________ Reaction:______________
Protein:_______________________ Glucose:_____________________ Acetone:_______________________________________

EXAMINATION AND INVESTIGATIONS

Blood Group:________ Rh Factor:_________ Hb:__________ VDRL:__________ HIV:__________Others:_______________
Heart_________ Lungs____________ Breast_____________ Abdomen_________________ Perineum___________________

DELIVERY RECORD

Onset of True Labour: Date:_______________ Time:__________________
Time of Full Dilatation: Date:______________________ Time:________________________
Membranes Ruptured at:_____________________ Spontaneous/Artificial: ______________ PROM:____________________

a. Delivery of Baby

Baby Born at:_________________ AM/PM, Male/Female:_____________ Mode of Delivery:_______________________
Condition of Baby: Active/Nonactive/Asphyxiated _______________ Apgar Score _____________________________
Treatment: ____

b. Delivery of Placenta and Membranes

Delivery at:________________ AM/PM
Spontaneously/Manually removed____
Type of placenta____
Placenta and membranes: Complete/Incomplete____
Weight _____________ Cord Length___________________ Any Abnormality___________________________
Total Blood Loss:____

c. Perineum

Intact___________ Episiotomy________________ Laceration_________________________ Repair__________________
Medications Given ____
____
____

d. Length of Labour

Mode of Delivery: ____

DURATION OF LABOUR

Progress of Labour	Date	Time	Total...... Hrs..... Min.....
Contraction Started			...... Hrs..... Min.....
Full Dilatation			
Delivery of Baby			...... Hrs..... Min.....
Delivery of Placenta			...... Hrs..... Min.....
Total Time Taken for Labour			

e. Condition of the Mother following Delivery

Pulse: ____________________BP:____________________ Uterus: Hard/Soft Vaginal bleeding: ____________________

Breastfeeding initiated at: ____

Perineum Scar: Healthy/Not healthy

CLINICAL CHART OF BABY

Date: Temperature:																	
°F	°C																
104.0	40																
103.1	39.5																
102.2	39																
101.3	38.5																
100.4	38																
99.5	37.5																
98.6	37																
97.7	36.5																
96.8	36																
Heart Rate																	
Respiration																	
Urine																	
Stool																	
Vomit																	
Jaundice																	
Weight																	
Remarks																	

CLINICAL CHART OF PUERPERIUM

Date: Temperature:																	
°F	°C																
104.0	40																
103.1	39.5																
102.2	39																
101.3	38.5																
100.4	38																
99.5	37.5																
98.6	37																
97.7	36.5																
96.8	36																
95.9	35.5																
Respiration																	
BP																	
Lochia																	
Urine																	
Motion																	
Fundus in cm																	

Sign of Supervisor **Sign of Student**

POSTNATAL CARE

Name:_______________ Age:_______ G, P, L, A _______________
Name of the Hospital:_______________ Hospital Number: _______________
Date of Delivery:_______________ Date of Discharge:_______________
Date of Registration:_______________ LMP: _______ EDD: _______________
Prenatal Record:_______________ Gestation at 1st visit: _______________

MEDICAL HISTORY

Chronic Illness:_______________
Surgery:_______________
Allergy:_______________
Communicable Disease:_______________

FAMILY HISTORY

Type of Family:
Nuclear:_______________ Number of Persons:_______________
Joint:_______________ Number of Persons:_______________

HISTORY OF MULTIPLE BIRTHS

Number of Children:_______________ Girl Child:_______________ Boy Child_______________

SOCIOECONOMIC BACKGROUND

Religion:_______________ Family Income:_______________
Education: Husband:_______________ Wife: _______________
Occupation: Husband: _______________ Wife: _______________

DISEASES: Chronic Illness: _______ Genetic Disorder: _______ Psychiatric Disorder:_______

MENSTRUAL HISTORY

Menarchy:_______________Duration:_______________Interval:_______________Flow:_______

MARITAL HISTORY

Age of marriage:_______________ Year of Marriage: _______________
Consanguineous: Yes/No

DIETARY PATTERN

Vegetarian:_______________ Nonvegetarian: _______________
Likes: _______________ Dislikes: _______________
Habits: Smoking/Drinking Alchohol/Chewing pan/Tobacco

PAST OBSTETRICAL HISTORY

S.No	Year	Full Term	Abortion	Type of Delivery	Sex of Baby	Alive	Stillbirth	Weight	Remarks

PRESENT PREGNANCY

Admission Notes:

Admission on:____________ at:____________ Contractions Commenced:____________ at:____________

Period of Gestation:____________ Membranes: Intact:____________ Ruptured on:____________

Involution of Uterus:____________ Contractions____________

Presentation:____________ Position:____________

Engaged/Nonengaged:____________ FHR:____________

Bladder:____________ Bowel:____________

BP:____________ TPR:____________

Special Observations:____________

PRENATAL VISITS

Date of Booking	Weight	Height	Urine		BP	FHR	Weeks of Gestation	Height of Fundus	Position	Treatment
			Protein	Glucose						

GENERAL CONDITION

BP:__________ TPR:____________________________ Urine: Sp. gavity___________________ Reaction:______________

Protein:_________________________ Glucose:_____________________ Acetone:____

EXAMINATION AND INVESTIGATIONS

Blood Group:________ Rh Factor:_________ Hb:__________ VDRL:__________ HIV:__________Others:_______________

Heart__________ Lungs_____________ Breast______________ Abdomen_________________ Perineum___________________

DELIVERY RECORD

Onset of True Labour: Date:________________ Time:___________________

Time of Full Dilatation: Date:________________________ Time:_________________________

Membranes Ruptured at:______________________ Spontaneous/Artificial: _______________ PROM:__________________

a. Delivery of Baby

Baby Born at:__________________ AM/PM, Male/Female:______________ Mode of Delivery:________________________

Condition of Baby: Active/Nonactive/Asphyxiated ________________ Apgar Score ________________________________

Treatment: ____

b. Delivery of Placenta and Membranes

Delivery at:________________ AM/PM

Spontaneously/Manually removed____

Type of placenta____

Placenta and membranes: Complete/Incomplete____

Weight ______________ Cord Length___________________ Any Abnormality____

Total Blood Loss:____

c. Perineum

Intact___________ Episiotomy________________ Laceration_________________________ Repair___________________

Medications Given ____

____

____

d. Length of Labour

Mode of Delivery: ____

DURATION OF LABOUR

Progress of Labour	Date	Time	Total...... Hrs..... Min.....
Contraction Started			...... Hrs..... Min.....
Full Dilatation			
Delivery of Baby			...... Hrs..... Min.....
Delivery of Placenta			...... Hrs..... Min.....
Total Time Taken for Labour			

e. Condition of the Mother following Delivery

Pulse: ________________BP:________________ Uterus: Hard/Soft Vaginal bleeding: ________________
Breastfeeding initiated at: ____
Perineum Scar: Healthy/Not healthy

CLINICAL CHART OF BABY

Date: Temperature:																	
°F	°C																
104.0	40																
103.1	39.5																
102.2	39																
101.3	38.5																
100.4	38																
99.5	37.5																
98.6	37																
97.7	36.5																
96.8	36																
Heart Rate																	
Respiration																	
Urine																	
Stool																	
Vomit																	
Jaundice																	
Weight																	
Remarks																	

CLINICAL CHART OF PUERPERIUM

Date: Temperature:																	
°F	°C																
104.0	40																
103.1	39.5																
102.2	39																
101.3	38.5																
100.4	38																
99.5	37.5																
98.6	37																
97.7	36.5																
96.8	36																
95.9	35.5																
Respiration																	
BP																	
Lochia																	
Urine																	
Motion																	
Fundus in cm																	

Sign of Supervisor **Sign of Student**

VAGINAL EXAMINATION

RECORD OF PER VAGINAL EXAMINATION

Name:____________________ Age:__________ Reg. No: ____________
G, P, L, A:________________ LMP:____________ EDD:____________
Gestational Age (wks): ____________________________________

STATUS OF VULVA

Condition of skin:____________________________
Discharge:________________________________
Edema: __________________________________
Infection:_________________________________

FINDING OF P/V EXAMINATION

Cervical Dilatation:____________________________

Cervical Effacement:___________________________

Sacral Promontory:____________________________

Membranes: ________________________________

Presentation:_______________________________

Presenting Part:_____________________________

Station: __________________________________

Show: ___________________________________

Moulding:_________________________________

Caput Succedaneum: ___________________________

Amniotic Fluid:______________________________

PERINEUM:________________________________

Sign of Supervisor **Sign of Student**

RECORD OF PER VAGINAL EXAMINATION

Name:____________________ Age:__________ Reg. No: __________

G, P, L, A:________________ LMP:______________ EDD:______________

Gestational Age (wks): ____________________

STATUS OF VULVA

Condition of skin:____________________

Discharge:____________________

Edema: ____________________

Infection:____________________

FINDING OF P/V EXAMINATION

Cervical Dilatation:____________________

Cervical Effacement:____________________

Sacral Promontory:____________________

Membranes: ____________________

Presentation:____________________

Presenting Part:____________________

Station: ____________________

Show: ____________________

Moulding:____________________

Caput Succedaneum: ____________________

Amniotic Fluid:____________________

PERINEUM:____________________

Sign of Supervisor **Sign of Student**

RECORD OF PER VAGINAL EXAMINATION

Name:______________________ Age:____________ Reg. No: ______________

G, P, L, A:__________________ LMP:______________ EDD:______________

Gestational Age (wks): ____

STATUS OF VULVA

Condition of skin:____________________________________

Discharge:____________________________________

Edema: ____________________________________

Infection:____________________________________

FINDING OF P/V EXAMINATION

Cervical Dilatation:____________________________________

Cervical Effacement:____________________________________

Sacral Promontory:____________________________________

Membranes: ____________________________________

Presentation:____________________________________

Presenting Part:____________________________________

Station: ____________________________________

Show: ____________________________________

Moulding:____________________________________

Caput Succedaneum: ____________________________________

Amniotic Fluid:____________________________________

PERINEUM:____________________________________

Sign of Supervisor **Sign of Student**

RECORD OF PER VAGINAL EXAMINATION

Name:________________ Age:________ Reg. No: __________

G, P, L, A:____________ LMP:__________ EDD:__________

Gestational Age (wks): ____________________

STATUS OF VULVA

Condition of skin:____________________

Discharge:____________________

Edema: ____________________

Infection:____________________

FINDING OF P/V EXAMINATION

Cervical Dilatation:____________________

Cervical Effacement:____________________

Sacral Promontory:____________________

Membranes: ____________________

Presentation:____________________

Presenting Part:____________________

Station: ____________________

Show: ____________________

Moulding:____________________

Caput Succedaneum: ____________________

Amniotic Fluid:____________________

PERINEUM:____________________

Sign of Supervisor **Sign of Student**

RECORD OF PER VAGINAL EXAMINATION

Name:______________________ Age:____________ Reg. No: ______________

G, P, L, A:________________ LMP:________________ EDD:________________

Gestational Age (wks): ____

STATUS OF VULVA

Condition of skin:________________________________

Discharge:________________________________

Edema: ________________________________

Infection:________________________________

FINDING OF P/V EXAMINATION

Cervical Dilatation:________________________________

Cervical Effacement:________________________________

Sacral Promontory:________________________________

Membranes: ________________________________

Presentation:________________________________

Presenting Part:________________________________

Station: ________________________________

Show: ________________________________

Moulding:________________________________

Caput Succedaneum: ________________________________

Amniotic Fluid:________________________________

PERINEUM:________________________________

Sign of Supervisor **Sign of Student**

EPISIOTOMY AND SUTURE

S.No.	Date	Reg. No.	Name of the Patient	Gravida	Para	Indication	Type of Episiotomy	Remarks	Supervisor Signature
1.									
2.									
3.									
4.									
5.									

NEONATAL RESUSCITATION

NEWBORN RESUSCITATION

Baby of:____________________ Sex of Baby:________________ Birth Weight:____________________

Date of Birth:________________ Time of Birth:____________________

BIRTH DETAILS

Term:____

Mode of Delivery: ____

Type of Labour: ____

Assistance Provided: ____

CONDITION OF NEWBORN AT BIRTH

Apgar Score: At 1 min: ____________________

At 5 min : ____________________

General Condition: ____

____

Cause of Poor Condition: ____

____

IMMEDIATE INTERVENTIONS DONE AFTER BIRTH

____

____

____

____

Drug Given (if any):____

____

Newborn Transfer to:____________________ Time:____________________

Sign of Supervisor **Sign of Student**

NEWBORN RESUSCITATION

Baby of:______________________ Sex of Baby:__________________ Birth Weight:______________________

Date of Birth:____________________ Time of Birth:________________________

BIRTH DETAILS

Term:____

Mode of Delivery: ____

Type of Labour: ____

Assistance Provided: ____

_

CONDITION OF NEWBORN AT BIRTH

Apgar Score: At 1 min: ________________________

At 5 min : ________________________

General Condition: ____

_

____

Cause of Poor Condition: ____

____

_

IMMEDIATE INTERVENTIONS DONE AFTER BIRTH

____

____

____

____

Drug Given (if any):____

____

Newborn Transfer to:____________________________ Time:________________________________

Sign of Supervisor **Sign of Student**

NEWBORN RESUSCITATION

Baby of:______________________ Sex of Baby:________________ Birth Weight:______________________

Date of Birth:__________________ Time of Birth:________________________

BIRTH DETAILS

Term:____

Mode of Delivery: ____
Type of Labour: ____
Assistance Provided: ____

CONDITION OF NEWBORN AT BIRTH

Apgar Score: At 1 min: ________________________
At 5 min : ________________________

General Condition: ____
____

Cause of Poor Condition: ____
____

IMMEDIATE INTERVENTIONS DONE AFTER BIRTH

____
____
____
____

Drug Given (if any):____
____

Newborn Transfer to:_____________________________ Time:___________________________________

Sign of Supervisor **Sign of Student**

NEWBORN RESUSCITATION

Baby of:__________ Sex of Baby:__________ Birth Weight:__________

Date of Birth:__________ Time of Birth:__________

BIRTH DETAILS

Term:__________

Mode of Delivery: __________
Type of Labour: __________
Assistance Provided: __________

CONDITION OF NEWBORN AT BIRTH

Apgar Score: At 1 min: __________
At 5 min : __________

General Condition: __________

Cause of Poor Condition: __________

IMMEDIATE INTERVENTIONS DONE AFTER BIRTH

____

Drug Given (if any):__________

Newborn Transfer to:__________ Time:__________

Sign of Supervisor **Sign of Student**

NEWBORN RESUSCITATION

Baby of:__________ Sex of Baby:__________ Birth Weight:__________

Date of Birth:__________ Time of Birth:__________

BIRTH DETAILS

Term:__________

Mode of Delivery: __________
Type of Labour: __________
Assistance Provided: __________

CONDITION OF NEWBORN AT BIRTH

Apgar Score: At 1 min: __________
At 5 min : __________

General Condition: __________

Cause of Poor Condition: __________

IMMEDIATE INTERVENTIONS DONE AFTER BIRTH

Drug Given (if any):__________

Newborn Transfer to:__________ Time:__________

Sign of Supervisor **Sign of Student**

ASSIST WITH CAESAREAN SECTION

Name:______________________ Age:__________ G, P, L, A______________
Name of the Hospital:__________________ Hospital Number:__________________
Date of Admission:____________________

ANTENATAL RECORD

Date of Booking:__________ LMP:________ EDD:________ Gestation at 1st Visit:__________

MEDICAL HISTORY

Chronic Illness:______________________________
Surgery:______________________________
Allergy: ______________________________
Communicable Disease: ______________________________

FAMILY HISTORY

Type of Family:
Nuclear:______________________ Number of Persons:______________
Joint:______________________ Number of Persons:______________

DISEASES: Chronic Illness

Hypertension: __________ Diabetes:__________ Genetic Diseases:________ Psychiatric Disorders:________
Others: ______________________________

HISTORY OF MULTIPLE BIRTHS

Socioeconomic Background:
Religion:__________________ Family Income:__________________
Education: Husband:__________________ Wife: __________________
Occupation: Husband: __________________ Wife: __________________

MENSTRUAL HISTORY

Menarchy:__________ Duration:__________ Interval:__________ Flow:__________

MARITAL HISTORY

Age of Marriage:______________
Consanguineous: Yes/No

DIETARY PATTERN

Vegetarian: __________________ Nonvegetarian: __________________
Likes: __________________ Dislikes: __________________
Habits: Smoking/Drinking Alcohol/Chewing Pan/Tobacco

PAST OBSTETRICAL HISTORY

S.No	Year	Full Term	Abortion	Type of Delivery	Sex of Baby	Alive	Stillbirth	Weight	Remarks

PRESENT PREGNANCY

Admission Notes:
Admission on:__________ at:______________ Contractions Commenced:___________ at:______________________
Period of Gestation:______________________ Membranes: Intact:________________ Ruptured on:_______________
Height of Fundus:______________________ Contractions____
Presentation: ___________________________ Position: ____
Engaged/Nonengaged: ___________________ FHR: ____
Bladder:_______________________________ Bowel:____
BP: __________________________________ TPR: ____
Special Observations: ____
Diagnosis of High-risk Status in Antenatal Period: ____

PRENATAL VISITS

Date of Booking	Weight	Height	Urine		BP	FHR	Weeks of Gestation	Height of Fundus	Position	Treatment
			Protein	Glucose						

EXAMINATION AND INVESTIGATIONS

Blood Group:________ Rh Factor:__________ Hb:____________ VDRL:________ HIV:_________ Others:_______________
Heart__________ Lungs_____________ Breast______________ Abdomen_____________ Perineum__________________

Indication for Caesarean Section:____
Type of Operation: ____
Type of Caesarean Section: ____
Preoperative Preparation Done:______________________________ Patient Shifted to OT at:_____________________

Operative Room Record

Anaesthesia Given:________________________ Type:________________ Drug: ________________________________

Baby Delivered at: ___________________________ AM/PM

Immediate Care for Newborn: ____

Delivery of Placenta and Membrane: ____

Suturing of Uterine and Abdominal Layers: ________________________________

Postoperative Care in Recovery Room

Mother: ____

____

Baby: ____

____

Postoperative Order

____

____

____

Transfer to Postnatal Ward: At____

Condition on transfer: Mother____

Sign of Supervisor **Sign of Student**

ASSISTED WITH CAESAREAN SECTION

Name:______________________ Age:__________ G, P, L, A__________
Name of the Hospital:______________ Hospital Number:______________
Date of Admission:______________

ANTENATAL RECORD

Date of Booking:__________ LMP:________ EDD:________ Gestation at 1st Visit:__________

MEDICAL HISTORY

Chronic Illness:______________________
Surgery:______________________
Allergy: ______________________
Communicable Disease: ______________________

FAMILY HISTORY

Type of Family:
Nuclear:______________________ Number of Persons:______________
Joint:______________________ Number of Persons:______________

DISEASES: Chronic Illness

Hypertension: __________Diabetes:________ Genetic Diseases:________ Psychiatric Disorders:________
Others: ______________________

HISTORY OF MULTIPLE BIRTHS

Socioeconomic Background:
Religion:______________ Family Income:______________
Education: Husband:______________ Wife: ______________
Occupation: Husband: ______________ Wife: ______________

MENSTRUAL HISTORY

Menarchy:__________Duration:________Interval:__________Flow:__________

MARITAL HISTORY

Age of Marriage:______________
Consanguineous: Yes/No

DIETARY PATTERN

Vegetarian: ______________ Nonvegetarian: ______________
Likes: ______________ Dislikes: ______________
Habits: Smoking/Drinking Alcohol/Chewing Pan/Tobacco

PAST OBSTETRICAL HISTORY

S.No	Year	Full Term	Abortion	Type of Delivery	Sex of Baby	Alive	Stillbirth	Weight	Remarks

PRESENT PREGNANCY

Admission Notes:
Admission on:__________ at: ______________ Contractions Commenced:____________ at:______________________
Period of Gestation:______________________ Membranes: Intact:_________________Ruptured on:______________
Height of Fundus:_______________________ Contractions____
Presentation: _________________________ Position: ____
Engaged/Nonengaged: __________________ FHR: ____
Bladder:_____________________________ Bowel:____
BP: _______________________________ TPR: ____
Special Observations: ____
Diagnosis of High-risk Status in Antenatal Period: ____

PRENATAL VISITS

Date of Booking	Weight	Height	Urine		BP	FHR	Weeks of Gestation	Height of Fundus	Position	Treatment
			Protein	Glucose						

EXAMINATION AND INVESTIGATIONS

Blood Group:________ Rh Factor:__________ Hb:____________ VDRL:________ HIV:_________Others:______________
Heart__________ Lungs_____________ Breast______________ Abdomen_____________ Perineum__________________

Indication for Caesarean Section:____
Type of Operation: ____
Type of Caesarean Section: ____
Preoperative Preparation Done:______________________________ Patient Shifted to OT at:________________________

Operative Room Record

Anaesthesia Given:________________________ Type:________________ Drug: ____________________________________

Baby Delivered at: ___________________________ AM/PM

Immediate Care for Newborn: ____

Delivery of Placenta and Membrane: ___________________________________

Suturing of Uterine and Abdominal Layers: _____________________________

Postoperative Care in Recovery Room

Mother: ____

____

Baby: ____

____

Postoperative Order

____

____

____

Transfer to Postnatal Ward: At____

Condition on transfer: Mother____

Sign of Supervisor **Sign of Student**

WITNESS/ASSIST ABNORMAL DELIVERIES

S. No.	Date	Reg. No.	Name of the Patient	G, P, L, A	LMP	EDD	Wks of Gestation	Presentation/ Position	Baby Sex/Wt.	Supervised by
1.										
2.										
3.										
4.										
5.										

INSERTION OF IUD

Name:_______________ Age:______ Reg. No:__________________ Religion:_____________________ Reg.No.______________
Date of Insertion:_________________G, P, L, A:_________________ LMP:___________________ EDD:________________
Address:_____________________________________Education:_________________Occupation:_________________________

HISTORY TAKING

Significant History of Women:____

OBSTETRIC HISTORY

No. of Children:__________________________ Boys:____________________ Girls:______________________
Age of Elder Issue:_________________________ Age of Last is_______________
Any Health Problem to Childrens:____

HEALTH EXAMINATION OF WOMEN

General:____

Pelvic:____

IUCD INSERTION

Time:____
Type: ____

PROCEDURE

Pre operative preparation:____

Interaoperative:____

Postoperative:____

Sign of Supervisor **Sign of Student**

INSERTION OF IUD

Name:__________ Age:_____ Reg. No:__________ Religion:__________ Reg. No.__________
Date of Insertion:__________ G, P, L, A:__________ LMP:__________ EDD:__________
Address:__________ Education:__________ Occupation:__________

HISTORY TAKING

Significant History of Women:__________

OBSTETRIC HISTORY

No. of Children:__________ Boys:__________ Girls:__________
Age of Elder Issue:__________ Age of Last is__________
Any Health Problem to Childrens:__________

HEALTH EXAMINATION OF WOMEN

General:__________

Pelvic:__________

IUCD INSERTION

Time:__________
Type: __________

PROCEDURE

Pre operative preparation:__________

Interaoperative:__________

Postoperative:__________

Sign of Supervisor **Sign of Student**

INSERTION OF IUD

Name:______________ Age:______ Reg. No:________________ Religion:____________________ Reg.No.____________
Date of Insertion:________________G, P, L, A:________________ LMP:__________________ EDD:________________
Address:__________________________________Education:_______________Occupation:________________________

HISTORY TAKING

Significant History of Women:____

OBSTETRIC HISTORY

No. of Children:________________________ Boys:____________________ Girls:______________________
Age of Elder Issue:_______________________ Age of Last is______________
Any Health Problem to Childrens:____

HEALTH EXAMINATION OF WOMEN

General:____

Pelvic:____

IUCD INSERTION

Time:____
Type: ____

PROCEDURE

Pre operative preparation:____

Interaoperative:____

Postoperative:____

Sign of Supervisor **Sign of Student**

INSERTION OF IUD

Name:______________ Age:______ Reg. No:_________________ Religion:____________________ Reg.No.______________
Date of Insertion:_________________G, P, L, A:_________________ LMP:__________________ EDD:__________________
Address:____________________________________Education:________________Occupation:_______________________

HISTORY TAKING

Significant History of Women:____
____
____
____

OBSTETRIC HISTORY

No. of Children:_________________________ Boys:____________________ Girls:______________________
Age of Elder Issue:________________________ Age of Last is______________
Any Health Problem to Childrens:____

HEALTH EXAMINATION OF WOMEN

General:____
____
____

Pelvic:____
____
____

IUCD INSERTION

Time:____
Type: ____

PROCEDURE

Pre operative preparation:____
____
____

Interaoperative:____
____
____

Postoperative:____
____
____

Sign of Supervisor **Sign of Student**

INSERTION OF IUD

Name:__________ Age:____ Reg. No:__________ Religion:__________ Reg.No.__________
Date of Insertion:__________ G, P, L, A:__________ LMP:__________ EDD:__________
Address:____________________ Education:__________ Occupation:__________

HISTORY TAKING

Significant History of Women:____________________

OBSTETRIC HISTORY

No. of Children:__________ Boys:__________ Girls:__________
Age of Elder Issue:__________ Age of Last is__________
Any Health Problem to Childrens:____________________

HEALTH EXAMINATION OF WOMEN

General:____________________

Pelvic:____________________

IUCD INSERTION

Time:____________________
Type:____________________

PROCEDURE

Pre operative preparation:____________________

Interaoperative:____________________

Postoperative:____________________

Sign of Supervisor **Sign of Student**

CHECKLIST

CHECKLIST FOR ASSESSMENT IN LABOUR

(HISTORY)

S.No	STEP	OBSERVATION
1.	Prepare the necessary equipment and introduce yourself	
2.	Give the woman a seat or a bed to lie on, depending on her condition	
3.	Help the woman onto the examination table and make her comfortable	
4.	Make an immediate assessment of whether delivery is imminent (pushing, grunting, bulging thin perineum, or vagina gaping and head visible)	
5.	Write identification data and record chief complain of women	
6.	Note following information and record her response: • When labour pains started • Whether she has noticed a trickle or gush of fluid (if so, when, how much and colour) • Frequency of labour pains • Intensity of labour pains • Presence of vaginal bleeding or bloody mucus (show) • Presence of foetal movement and whether it is normal or changed • When was the last time she passed urine and stools when did she last eat • If she took any medicine or treatment to speed up or slow down labour and whether they worked	
7.	Check the woman's antenatal record for her (H/O previous delivery, Present investigation, vaccine, any medical problem, HIV Status if any)	
8.	Calculate the expected date of delivery and gestational age	

CHECKLIST FOR GENERAL EXAMINATION IN LABOUR

S.No	STEPS	OBSERVATION
1.	• Prepare the necessary equipment • Antenatal assessment tray	
2.	Wash hands thoroughly with soap and water and air dry them	
3.	Explain each step of the physical examination to the woman. The woman should be made comfortable.	
4.	Take the woman's blood pressure, pulse and temperature: • Check her height and general appearance (whether she is looking ill, exhausted or malnourished) • Record your findings	
5.	Check the woman's conjunctiva, tongue and palms for pallor and hydration state	
6.	Count the respiratory rate and note the kind of breathing (normal, shallow, deep, gasping) between and during contractions, count the heart rate	
7.	Look for enlarged neck veins and shortness of breath which may mean serious sickness	
8.	Look and feel the breasts for problems that might interfere with breastfeeding	
9.	Look and feel the arms and legs for swelling	
10.	Look for deformities of legs, back and pelvis that may make vaginal delivery difficult or impossible	
11.	Recording of specific findings	

CHECKLIST FOR ABDOMINAL EXAMINATION IN LABOUR

S.No	STEPS	OBSERVATION
1.	Prepare the necessary things, maintain privacy of patient: • Examination bed • Foetoscope • Client's records with partograph • Watch with seconds hand	
2.	Explain before the steps of procedure in detail and answer women and relative enquire	
	ABDOMINAL EXAMINATION	
1.	Ask the woman if she needs to empty her bladder. (Save urine for testing, if necessary.)	
2.	Help the woman on to the examination table and relax the women with some deep breathing.	
3.	Wash hands thoroughly with soap and water	
4.	Explain each step of the abdominal examination as you proceed	
5.	Observe shape and size of the abdomen and presence of scars. Look for the way the baby is lying and its movements, contractions, unusual shapes, estimating fundal height.	
6.	Press gently and move hand down the abdomen until the curved upper border of the fundus is felt. Use landmarks of the umbilicus and sternum to help confirm fundal height.	
	DETERMINING LIE AND PRESENTATION	
1.	Face the woman's head. Stand on the right side	
2.	Place your hands on the sides of the fundus and curve fingers around top of fundus. • Feel for contraction. • Hold hands in the same position for the entire contraction of the uterus • Feel the strength of the contraction. • Time the duration of the contraction.	
3.	Between contractions, palpate shape, size, consistency and mobility: • The foetal breech will feel irregular, larger or bulkier than a head; the breech cannot be well outlined or readily moved or balloted. • The foetal head feels round and hard and can be balloted between your hands or between the thumb and a finger of one hand. • If there is a transverse lie, the fundus (suprapubic region) will feel empty.	
4.	Now place one hand on either side of the uterus about halfway between the symphysis pubis and the fundus: • The foetal back will feel like a firm, curved, continuously smooth mass extending from the breech to the neck. If you cannot feel the back on either side, then the back is towards the back of the woman, a posterior position. In a transverse lie the baby's body is felt across the abdomen.	
5.	Apply pressure to one side of the uterus, pushing the foetus to the other side of the abdomen against your other hand (your examining hand).	
6.	Palpates the other side of the uterus, from the abdominal midline to the lateral side and from the symphysis pubis to the fundus: • The foetal hands, feet, knees and elbows will feel small, knobby and irregular and will move when pressed on.	
7.	Reverse the procedure to examine the other side of the uterus, using the other hand as the examining hand and pressing with the hand used for examination on the other side.	
8.	Now use the thumb and four fingers to grasp the portion of the lower abdomen immediately above the symphysis pubis.	
9.	Press gently but firmly into the abdomen to feel the presenting part below and between your thumb and four fingers.	
10.	Palpate for shape, size, consistency and mobility to determine the head or the breech: • If the presenting part is the head, try to move it from side to side. If the head cannot be moved it is engaged. • If neither the head nor the buttocks are felt, the baby is lying sideways, a transverse presentation.	
11.	Now turn and face the woman's feet. Make sure that the woman still has her knees bent.	

S.No	STEPS	OBSERVATION
12.	Place one hand on either side of the uterus with the palms just below the level of the umbilicus and fingers directed toward the symphysis pubis.	
13.	Press deeply with fingertips into the lower abdomen and move them toward the pelvic inlet: • A vertex presentation is indicated if one hand feels the sinciput (hard round mass) on the same side of the abdomen that the foetal small parts were felt, while at the same time the other hand continues down toward the pelvis. • A breech presentation is indicated if both hands continue to move toward the pelvic inlet and experience a feeling of "give" along with the trunk of the foetus. • In transverse lie, no pole is felt • Feel to assess if there is more than one baby	
	ASSESSING DESCENT OF THE FOETAL HEAD	
14.	Feel the presenting part with your right hand. Place the fingers of the other hand horizontally above the symphysis pubis and see how much of the head can be felt above it: • 5 finger breadths = 5/5 (five-fifths) above the brim • 4 finger breadths = 4/5 (four-fifths) above the brim • 3 finger breadths = 3/5 (three-fifths) above the brim • 2 finger breadths = 2/5 (two-fifths) above the brim (the head is generally accepted to be engaged when the portion above the pelvic brim is represented by two fingers). Verify findings on vaginal exam.	
	CHECKING UTERINE CONTRACTIONS	
15.	Ask the woman to lie on her left side. Place your hand on the woman's abdomen to feel the contractions.	
16.	Palpate the number of contractions in a 10-minute period, time their duration in seconds and assess the strength. Record your findings.	
	FOETAL MOVEMENT/FHR	
20.	Ask if the baby is moving regularly and observe for foetal movement during the examination.	
21.	Place the foetoscope on the woman's abdomen at right angles to it immediately following a contraction. For vertex and breech presentations listen through the back of the foetus.	
22.	Count the heart rate for one full minute (while listening to the foetal heart, the hand should not touch the foetoscope).	

CHECKLIST FOR VAGINAL EXAMINATION IN LABOUR

S.No	STEPS	OBSERVATION
1.	Ask the woman to flex her knees and separate her legs. Ensure that the bladder is empty and the woman does not have a desire to pass urine.	
2.	Cleanse the vulva from above downwards with one gloved hand (not the examining hand), using a swab dipped in an antiseptic solution.	
	EXAMINING THE VAGINA	
1.	The vaginal opening is clearly visualised. Once your fingers are inserted do not take them out till the examination is complete.	
2.	Direct the fingers along the anterior wall of the vagina and note: • Vaginal temperature and moisture (should be warm and moist) • Vaginal texture (should be soft and distensible) • Feel for hard scarring and stool in the rectum	
	EXAMINING THE CERVIX	
1.	Keep the other hand (abdominal hand) on the client's abdomen in the suprapubic region. When the examining fingers reach the end of vagina, turn the pads of the fingers upwards to come in contact with the cervix. You will be able to feel and examine the cervix.	
2.	Palpate around the fornices and sense the proximity of the presenting part of the foetus to the examining fingers.	
3.	Gently sweep the fingers from side to side to locate the cervical os: This will be felt as an opening in the cervix. • The os is normally situated centrally but sometimes in early labour it will be very posterior (backwards).	

S.No	STEPS	OBSERVATION
4.	Note the length of the cervix: • A long, tightly closed cervix indicates that labour has not yet started. • Check for degree of effacement of the cervix	
5.	Feel the consistency of the cervix: • It should be soft and elastic and applied closely to the presenting part. • Note any hard scarring on the cervix which may affect cervical dilatation.	
6.	Measure dilatation of the cervical os by estimating the distance in centimeters between the two examining fingers: • Practise estimating cervical dilatation with cut-out rings during your free time. • 0 cm equates to a closed external cervical os • 10 cm equates to a full dilatation	
7.	Feel the application of the cervix to the presenting part: • When the presenting part is not well applied to the cervix, dilatation may not occur as efficiently as if the presenting part is well applied. • When the presenting part is not well applied to the cervix, it may mean that there is cephalopelvic disproportion. • Intact membranes can be felt through the dilating os. • If the membranes have ruptured, ensure that the colour of the amniotic fluid is clear and cord has not prolapsed.	
8.	Identify the presentation: • In vertex presentations (96% of cases), the hard bones of the vault of the skull will be felt. Feel for caput and moulding and how far the head has progressed in the cervix • A breech presentation means the buttocks or legs are at the cervix • A transverse presentation will present as an arm or shoulder at the cervix.	
9.	Inform the woman of findings and provide reassurance. Record all findings from the vaginal examination.	
10.	Monitor labour and record your findings on the partograph.	

CHECKLIST FOR ASSISTING A BIRTH

S.No	STEPS	OBSERVATION
1.	Provide comfortable position, do handwashing, reassure the patient explain the procedure. Wear the sterile gloves.	
2.	Use one hand to cover the perineum with a warm, moist pad for support to facilitate flexion and prevent perineal tears.	
3.	Place fingers of the other hand on the advancing head as the head is crowning.	
4.	After crowning (the head does not go up in the vagina after a contraction), allow the head to gradually extend under your hand	
5.	Gently Feel Around the Baby's Neck for the Cord: • If found, slacken the cord to form a loop through which the shoulders can pass. • If the cord is tightly wound around the neck, clamp the cord with two artery forceps, placed 3 cm apart, and cut the cord between the two clamps.	
6.	Allow restitution and external rotation of the head to occur. Clean the mouth and nose with sterile gauze pieces	
7.	Place one hand on either side of the baby's head, over the ears and ask the woman to push gently. Apply gentle downward traction to allow the anterior shoulder to slip beneath the symphysis pubis.	
8.	When the axillary crease is seen, guide the head and trunk in an upward curve to allow the posterior shoulder to escape over the perineum. Grasp the baby around the chest to aid the birth of the trunk and lift the baby toward the woman's abdomen. Note the time of delivery.	
9.	Immediate care of baby: Dry the baby quickly and thoroughly with a clean, dry towel/cloth immediately after birth. Wipe the baby's eyes from inner to outer side with two separate clean pieces of cloth/gauze piece.	

S.No	STEPS	OBSERVATION
10.	Observe the baby's breathing while completing steps 1 and 2: • If the baby is not breathing, clear the airway with the mucous extractor. If still the baby does not breathe begin resuscitation measures with bag and mask. If the baby is breathing normally, continue with the following care.	
11.	Clamping and Cutting the Cord : • Put the sterile ties tightly on the cord 2 cms. and 5 cms. from the baby's abdomen. • Cut the cord after 2-3 minutes of the birth, using a new blade. • Cut off the excess cord. Do not apply anything on the cut surface or the stump.	
12.	Note the Apgar Score of the baby. Weight the baby	
13.	Proceed for separation of the placenta	

CHECKLIST FOR ASSISTING A BIRTH:

ACTIVE MANAGEMENT OF THE THIRD STAGE OF LABOUR

S.No	STEPS	OBSERVATION
1.	Place one hand on the symphysis pubis and verify that the placenta has separated by pushing the uterus up from below : • Find the lower part of the uterus • Put your hand just above the symphysis pubis, and push the uterus up from below • Look to see if the cord moves up with the uterus • If the cord does not move up, the placenta is probably separated • If the cord moves up with the uterus, the placenta is probably still attached, wait and try again later.	
2.	If the cord does not move up when pushing the uterus up, the placenta is probably separated - deliver the placenta	
3.	When the placenta is visible at the vaginal opening, cup it in both hands. Use a gentle upward and downward movement or twisting action to deliver the membranes. Place the placenta in basin.	
4.	Check complete placenta or its membrane are present or not. Gently massage the uterus and make sure that the uterus is well contracted.	
5.	If the placenta does not come out in 10 to 15 minutes after giving tab. Misoprostol and the woman is not bleeding, try and remove the placenta again by CCT.	
6.	Encourage the woman urinate. A full bladder can slow the birth of the placenta. Encourage her to breast feed her baby.	
7.	If the placenta is still not delivered after 30 minutes and the woman is not bleeding excessively, ask the woman to lie on her back. Explain that you will put your hand in her vagina to feel if the placenta has separated but is sitting in the vagina or cervix	
8.	Your non-examining hand should be placed at the uterine fundus, to support the uterus. Grasp the cord with your examining hand and gently follow it up until just past the vagina to find out if the placenta is in the vagina and can be easily removed.	
9.	Deliver the placenta and membranes: • Hold the placenta in your examining hand and gently pull it out of the vagina • Deliver the placenta slowly, holding and supporting it with both hands • To deliver the membranes, hold the placenta in both hands, turn it slowly and gently, until the membranes are twisted. Then slowly and gently pull the membranes out.	
10.	Gently massage the uterus and make sure that the uterus is well contracted. If the placenta has not separated after 30 minutes of tab. Misoprostol and CCT, refer to 'checklist for identification and management of immediate and delayed postpartum haemorrhage' and manage accordingly.	

CHECKLIST FOR CARE IN THE IMMEDIATE POSTPARTUM PERIOD

S. No	STEPS	OBSERVATION
1.	Check the bladder, and assist the woman to void urine if full. If not empty the bladder.	
2.	Monitor vaginal bleeding, uterine fundus, vital signs, temperature, pulse and blood pressure: (After delivery of placenta check vaginal bleeding) every 5 minutes until uterus is well-contracted round and hard. • Every 10 minutes for the first 30 minutes after delivery • Then every 30 mins for the next three (3) hours • Then at least every 6–8 hours (3–4 times a day)	
3.	Keep the mother and the newborn together. Encourage and facilitate breastfeeding after 1 hour of birth, adequate fluid intake, good hygiene, frequent voiding of urine and rest.	
4.	Do complete examination of the baby and provide immediate care for the newborn, check: • Vital Signs (temperature, pulse, BP, and respirations) • Uterine fundus and contraction • Vaginal bleeding • Perineum	
5.	Give woman-centred counselling on postpartum care: • Rest • Nutrition • Resumption of sexual activity and safer sex • Hygiene • Breastfeeding	
6.	Provide counselling about family planning and provide contraception, if appropriate.	
7.	Examine the newborn for breathing, bleeding from the umbilicus and breastfeeding. Advise the mother to keep the baby warm and keep the nappy area clean and dry.	
8.	Discuss danger signals as written below and help the woman and her family develop a complication readiness plan for the newborn and the woman • Bleeding more than a heavy period or passing clots • Soft uterus that won't get hard with massaging • Abdominal pain • Fever • Urinary incontinence	
9.	Follow up-Discharge the woman (not before 24 hours postpartum). Schedule a postnatal visit within the first week on day 3 of delivery.	

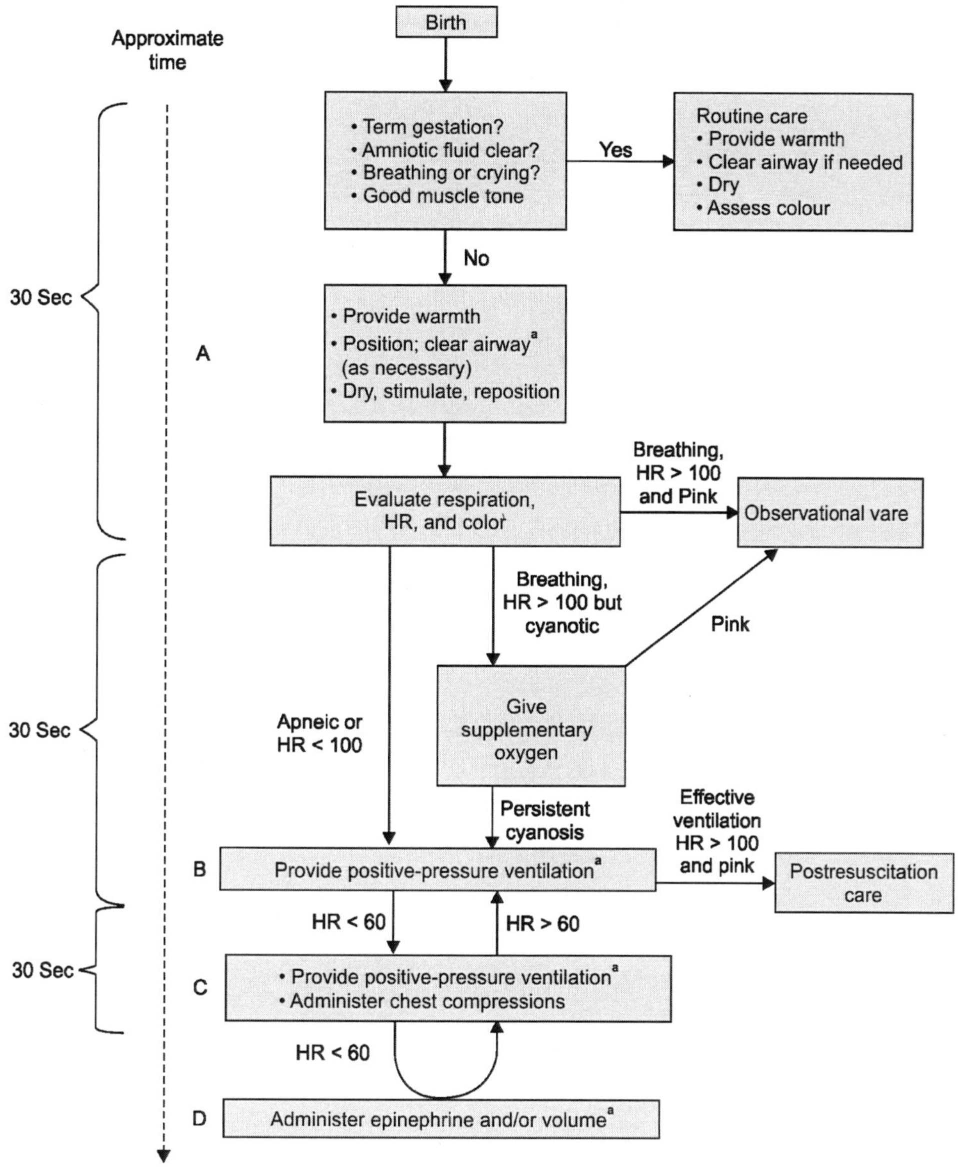

Approximate time
Birth
• Term gestation?
• Amniotic fluid clear?
• Breathing or crying?
• Good muscle tone
Yes
Routine care
• Provide warmth
• Clear airway if needed
• Dry
• Assess colour
No
30 Sec
A
• Provide warmth
• Position; clear airway[a] (as necessary)
• Dry, stimulate, reposition
Evaluate respiration, HR, and color
Breathing, HR > 100 and Pink
Observational vare
Breathing, HR > 100 but cyanotic
Pink
30 Sec
Apneic or HR < 100
Give supplementary oxygen
Persistent cyanosis
Effective ventilation HR > 100 and pink
B
Provide positive-pressure ventilation[a]
Postresuscitation care
HR < 60
HR > 60
30 Sec
C
• Provide positive-pressure ventilation[a]
• Administer chest compressions
HR < 60
D
Administer epinephrine and/or volume[a]